Community Care, Secondary Health Care and Care Management

Edited by
DAVID CHALLIS
ROBIN DARTON
KAREN STEWART

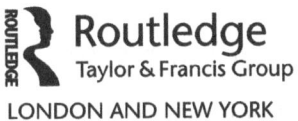
Routledge
Taylor & Francis Group

LONDON AND NEW YORK

First published 1998 by Ashgate Publishing

Reissued 2018 by Routledge
2 Park Square, Milton Park, Abingdon, Oxon, OX14 4RN
711 Third Avenue, New York, NY 10017

Routledge is an imprint of the Taylor & Francis Group, an informa business

Notice:
Product or corporate names may be trademarks or registered trademarks, and are used only for identification and explanation without intent to infringe.

Publisher's Note
The publisher has gone to great lengths to ensure the quality of this reprint but points out that some imperfections in the original copies may be apparent.

Disclaimer
The publisher has made every effort to trace copyright holders and welcomes correspondence from those they have been unable to contact.

A Library of Congress record exists under LC control number: 98073022

Typeset by Jane Dennett at the PSSRU, University of Kent at Canterbury

ISBN 13: 978-1-138-32142-7 (hbk)
ISBN 13: 978-1-138-32144-1 (pbk)
ISBN 13: 978-0-429-45253-6 (ebk)

Contents

List of Contributors

Ken Buckingham Health Economist, Cornwall and Isles of Scilly District and Family Health Services Authorities

Iain Carpenter Senior Lecturer in Health Care of the Elderly, King's College School of Medicine and Dentistry and Centre for Health Services Studies, University of Kent at Canterbury

Peter Carr Consultant Physician, Department of Geriatric Medicine, Darlington Memorial Hospital

David Challis Professor of Social Work and Community Care, Personal Social Services Research Unit, School of Psychiatry and Behavioural Sciences, University of Manchester, and University of Kent at Canterbury

Robin Darton Research Fellow, Personal Social Services Research Unit, University of Kent at Canterbury

Peter Huxley Professor of Psychiatric Social Work, School of Psychiatry and Behavioural Sciences, University of Manchester

Sally Ann Kelly Senior Occupational Therapist, Darlington Memorial Hospital

Christine McKee Project Leader, Eldercare Unit, Cornwall Healthcare Trust, Barncoose Hospital, Redruth, Cornwall

Douglas MacMahon Consultant Physician and Medical Director, Eldercare Unit, Cornwall Healthcare Trust, Barncoose Hospital, Redruth, Cornwall

Jackie Morris Consultant Physician in Old Age Medicine, Royal Free Hospital, London

Karen Stewart (Formerly Karen Traske) Research Officer, Personal Social Services Research Unit, University of Kent at Canterbury

Bob Welch Formerly Inspector, Social Care Group – Central Region, Social Services Inspectorate, Department of Health

Ken Wright Formerly Deputy Director, Centre for Health Economics, University of York

Preface

This book has grown out of the study of the Darlington Community Care Project. The Darlington Project was a special intervention funded under the Care in the Community Initiative, designed to provide frail elderly people with enhanced home care as an alternative to long-stay hospital care. The service consisted of care managers with budgets and control over multipurpose home care assistants who could act as assistants to nurses and therapy staff, and perform home care tasks in people's own homes. The project was one of the PSSRU family of care management projects evaluating intensive care management in a variety of settings, in this case a geriatric multidisciplinary team.

Following the publication of the book *Care Management and Health Care of Older People*, a conference was held at which the papers included in this book were presented. A key theme arising from the project and the conference is the role of secondary health care services in the provision of community care, and their link to intensive care management. We are particularly grateful to all those who presented the material in this book, and who have responded so generously to our editorial suggestions. The organisation of the conference itself would have not been possible without the painstaking hard work of Anne Walker and Glenys Harrison.

The manuscript has been typeset and edited by Jane Dennett at the PSSRU, and the diagrams were prepared by Nick Brawn at the PSSRU. We are grateful to the NHS Health Advisory Service for permission to reproduce (with amendments) a figure from their 1994 publication, *Comprehensive Health Services for Elderly People*, which appears as Figure 6.1 in Chapter 6. The appendices in Chapter 7 are reproduced from the *RAI-Home Care (RAI-HC) Assessment Manual*, by Morris et al., interRAI Corporation, Washington, DC, 1997. We should also like to thank the Department of Health and Ruth Chadwick, our liaison officer, for their support, and Professor Bleddyn Davies, the Director of the PSSRU, for his commitment to, and enthusiasm for, the research process.

David Challis, Robin Darton, Karen Stewart (formerly Traske), April 1998

1 Introduction

David Challis, Robin Darton and Karen Stewart

Community care has been a longstanding policy objective in the UK for all client groups. However, despite this formal commitment, a rapid growth in the residential and nursing home sectors during the 1980s, supported by social security funds, led to a perverse incentive towards institutional care (Audit Commission, 1986). The Government appointed a special adviser to identify possible solutions, and the report was published in 1988 (Griffiths, 1988). This recommended a more coordinated approach to the funding and management of care, placing the responsibility for the allocation of funds, assessment of need and co-ordination of care with the local authority social services department, and proposed care management to ensure a more effective use of resources. After this lengthy gestation period, the community care reforms in the UK emerged following the 1989 White Paper *Caring for People* (Cm 849, 1989) and the 1990 National Health Service and Community Care Act. Full implementation commenced in 1993. Underlying this change in policy were a set of six key objectives for service delivery:

- to promote the development of domiciliary, day and respite services to enable people to live in their own homes wherever feasible and sensible.
- to ensure that service providers make practical support for carers a high priority.

- to make proper assessment of need and good case management the cornerstone of high quality care.
- to promote the development of a flourishing independent sector alongside good quality public services.
- to clarify the responsibilities of agencies and so make it easier to hold them to account for their performance.
- to secure better value for taxpayers' money by introducing a new funding structure for social care.
  (Cm 849, 1989, para. 1.11.)

Much of the early activity was focused upon the establishment of organisational systems and funding arrangements, so as to provide an infrastructure for the operation of the new policy. Inevitably, much effort was focused upon these organisational arrangements, with a relative neglect of longer-term goals and development of the quality of agency practice. This book looks beyond the issues of early implementation by addressing several of the areas which provide real opportunities for effective service development. These areas include: finer differentiation of care management; links between assessment, care management and secondary health care; development of rehabilitation in the community; enhanced and more standardised assessment; and a degree of vertical integration of health and social care (that is, bringing together the relevant different service inputs required by specific client groups, for example people suffering from dementia).

Assessment and care management were identified as the cornerstones of this process of change, with the lead responsibility for effecting these activities being given to local authority social services departments. Since 1993, local authorities have invested a considerable amount of effort both in developing the procedures and processes for assessment and in developing a range of systems of care management. In their reviews of early developments following the implementation of the 1990 Act, the Social Services Inspectorate identified a number of concerns about both assessment and care management (Department of Health, 1993, 1994), which remain salient. The studies were intended to identify examples of good practice and to examine areas where developmental activity was required. The study on assessment procedures was undertaken during 1993 (Department of Health, 1993), and found a great deal of variation in both the content and the quality of the assessment documentation. Needs and problems tended to be categorised in a variety of ways, with a tendency to focus upon description rather than an analysis of need. The information collected appeared to lack both reliability and validity, and the lack of health care input was particularly evident. Local studies have also noted the need for there to be a more explicit link between the domains which require assessment, and the presence or accessibility of the requisite knowledge, skills and training to undertake that assessment effectively (Caldock, 1993). Analyses of the content of assessment documents have also noted a principal focus on functional domains, with a relative neglect of other areas (Caldock, 1994; Challis et al., 1996). The latter study examined, in detail, some 50 comprehensive assessment documents from a range of different local authorities, to examine the extent to which these documents covered the domains necessary for effective assessment. The only area in which more detailed and structured information was regularly recorded related to the performance of activities of daily living. Other factors such as continence, cognition, depressed mood, behavioural patterns or carer needs were covered more cursorily, if at all. Only a small minority of the assessment tools were jointly used by health and social care agencies, and the degree of variability of these assessment tools was high, with low comparability between them. The study of care management (Department of Health, 1994) also raised some concerns about development. These included a lack of differentiation of forms of care management, with considerable development of generic models of care management, and an extensive focus of activity upon short-term assessment, with insufficient time devoted to review. There was a lack of explicit linkage between care management arrangements and health care provision, with the exception of hospital discharge. Arrangements which formally linked long-term care approaches to care management and other services dealing with the more severely ill or dependent were not evident.

These concerns about developments within assessment and care management can be seen as linked. The lack of provision of specialist health care input to the assessment process, particularly at the point of transition from community-based care to nursing or residential care settings, also leads to problems at the time of review, when skills relevant to rehabilitation are also lacking. With regard to care management, concern has been expressed about the lack of differentiation between care management as a generic process and more intensive models of care management, focused upon more vulnerable and high-risk groups (Challis, 1994). On the one hand, there is a need for specialist health care input to meet complex needs and to facilitate critical decisions about placement, and, on the other, a need for a more specialised level of care management, or intensive care management, for more complex or high-need cases. The latter could be described as akin to the provision of secondary services in health care, whereas the more generic forms of care management, the first level of response, are more akin to primary health care. Likewise, specialist assessment skills could be seen as being located in secondary health care services. Despite this concordance of some of the requirements for effective community care and the changes which are occurring in secondary health care towards community-based modes of working, such as in geriatric medicine (British Geriatrics Society, 1994) and old age psychiatry (Dening, 1992), there has been relatively little such development in practice. This may, in part, be attributable to a preference for local developments rather than national direction, and the lack of a prescribed role within community care policies for secondary health care services. This may be contrasted with the parallel changes which occurred in Australia, which are described in Chapter 4.

The chapters in this book explore further the implications of a closer relationship between secondary health care services and care management, and how a number of areas of concern might be profitably addressed by facilitating new forms of linkages between the two. This book arose from a conference following the publication of *Care Management and Health Care of Older People* (Challis et al., 1995). This was a detailed evaluation of the Darlington Community Care Project, a care management service model located in a geriatric multidisciplinary team which provided intensive home care to frail older people as an alternative to long-stay hospital care. As such, it constitutes one of the few examples of linking care management and secondary health care. Another example which focused on older people with dementia and their carers is the Lewisham Intensive Case Management Scheme. This provided a case management service for people with dementia and their carers in a community mental health team for older people (Murphy and Challis, 1993; Challis et al., 1997).

In Chapter 2, Bob Welch explores some of the differences in the way care management has evolved in the UK following the community care reforms, and identifies four areas where further development is required. These are: the use of terminology; the nature and interpretation of the purchaser/provider separation; commissioning arrangements and delegation of responsibility; and the relationship between social work and care management. He identifies the considerable activity that has been undertaken and indicates the growing need for differentiation between the care management arrangements within an authority. One facet of this is the targeting of the most qualified and expert personnel to the appropriate level of need, which is seen as essential for successful implementation of care management. For example, for very dependent people this may require the development of intensive care management, dealing with a relatively small proportion of the cases who receive social care services, and linking with secondary health care services to provide some of the necessary expertise in assessment, care planning and rehabilitation.

In Chapter 3, Jackie Morris outlines the demographic and social changes which will affect the demand for services. In the context of an ageing population, cardio-vascular disease, osteoarthritis and accidental injuries are common causes of need for health care, along with the psychiatric problems of dementia and depressive disorders. The growing focus upon a primary care-led NHS has been coupled with a trend towards more acute and rehabilitation-focused services in geriatric medicine and old age psychiatry, organised around multidisciplinary teams. However, it is not entirely clear how these developments in secondary services mesh with primary care. One problem arising from the transfer of activity towards primary care is that the majority of general practitioners lack knowledge and training in geriatric medicine and mental health problems in old age. In a similar vein, despite the new community care arrangements, much of the activity provided by social care services is monodisciplinary. One solution towards which these factors point is the need for multidisciplinary teams with specialist expertise working in the community.

Chapter 4 reviews the main findings of the Darlington study, a care management initiative based in a geriatric multidisciplinary team, and suggests some of the organisational and service implications arising from it. It was one of a series of evaluations of intensive care management in varying settings for vulnerable older people. The Darlington study indicated that it was possible to offer a cost-effective, community-based intensive home support service for physically frail elderly people delivered through care management. The implic ations for policy and practice which were identified reflect the need to achieve better linkages between health and social care, and the potential advantages to be gained from linking secondary health care services into community-based care. Four factors are stressed: first, the integration of health and social care at the level of the hands-on worker, covering not just the boundary between community nursing and home care but also the link with paramedical and rehabilitative services; second, assessment, care management and secondary health care, in particular the currently unrecognised complementarity of functions; third, the nature of care management in a specialist setting, in particular its relevance to the development of intensive care management; and fourth, the location of care management services, including the advantages of location in a health care setting providing the environment for multidisciplinary assessment.

The history of moving innovatory services into mainstream provision indicates only too clearly the difficulties which need to be addressed if the benefits of the new are not to be submerged within the pre-existing broader pattern of activity (Fairweather et al., 1974; Backer et al., 1986; Ferlie et al., 1989). Chapter 5 discusses some of these in the context of the evolution of the Darlington service, and indicates some of the difficulties and disincentives which can occur when provision is shared between acute and community trusts. Such difficulties are likely to be exacerbated as continuing care becomes an unattractive area of activity for NHS trusts, where the critical boundary is with social care. The changes which Peter Carr and Sally Ann Kelly describe are a local manifestation of national debates about boundaries between agencies and units of provision. They raise the question of whether these disincentives and boundaries can only be overcome by the creation of a single budget for health and social services.

In Chapter 6, Doug MacMahon and his colleagues describe a pioneering service which offers a means whereby specialised health care activities, normally offered at a secondary level, can be provided in a community setting. Their study indicates that linking assessment with rehabilitation in this way may reduce carer stress and the probability of institutional placement. They conclude that specialist health assessment and rehabilitation have a particularly important role for people on the threshold of institutional care, those for whom discharge from hospital is likely to prove difficult, and direct referrals from general practitioners of people with ill health who wish to remain in their own homes.

In Chapter 7, Iain Carpenter outlines some of the difficulties in operationalising a more standard approach to assessment which can be used in both health and social care settings and become part of routine practice. The desirability of such an approach is seen as contrasting with the vague and imprecise documentation in much current practice, described earlier in this chapter, and offering a more purposive approach by linking assessment to care planning. He describes a recently developed approach for home care, the RAI-HC, which is based on the principles of the US Minimum Data Set for nursing homes (see Challis et al., 1996). He concludes that there is considerable opportunity for using a standard assessment across health and social care to improve skills and enhance the quality of assessments of frail older people so as to improve quality of care.

In Chapter 8, Peter Huxley considers the traditional distinctions between primary, secondary and tertiary levels of care and their utility for modern community care, based upon the experience of mental health services. In mental health care, with the current emphasis upon the effective treatment and management of severe mental illness, it is necessary to avoid placing too much emphasis upon primary health care alone. Moving secondary health care into the primary setting appears to confer some benefits, but still fails to address some structural disincentives for more integrated care. He suggests that, in addition, factors such as integrated management and budgeting, effective targeting, clinical rather than administrative case management, and establishing effective authority for case managers are important contributory factors. Some of these link with observations by Morris, and Carr and Kelly in earlier chapters.

In Chapter 9, Ken Wright discusses the complexity of cost relationships between hospital and community services, according to the levels of need of individuals. He then identifies issues which foster or impede the cost effectiveness of home-based care. These include: ensuring that investment in domiciliary care is paid for by savings in secondary care, which may involve investment in parallel services while the shift from

institutional to community care is made; the need for clarity of responsibility for the provision of domiciliary care, so that the possibilities for
substitution of more costly by less costly modes of provision, such as
home care instead of nursing, may be considered; clarity of access to
services and appropriate assessment; and interagency cooperation and
purchasing agreements. He also discusses the possibility of vertical
integration of care of older people, albeit fraught with difficulty because
of the number of organisations involved. He suggests that moves in
this direction might arise from initiatives such as programme budgeting
techniques, the development of multiprofessional community teams
and joint commissioning.

Chapter 10 brings together some of the key messages which recur
through this book. Possible solutions are identified through the recon-
figuration of services and other developments. These include the
growing importance of rehabilitation; the need for further work around
assessment processes and more standard, reliable approaches; and the
importance of addressing the more structural features of funding
between health and social care, which act to inhibit the development
of effective linkages between social care and secondary health care.
Included in this is a move towards vertical integration of care through
pooling of budgets and single commissioning strategies.

One factor which clearly emerges is that care management needs to
be developed differentially in the light of the different needs of different
user groups, different levels of need and local organisational circumstances. There is considerable room for further experimentation in the
redefinition of service roles and boundaries between health and social
care. This book attempts to clarify some of the developments which
the redefinition of service boundaries will require, if we are to provide
more effective community-based care and maintain access to specialist
skills as the locus of care provision shifts.

References

Audit Commission (1986) *Making a Reality of Community Care*, HMSO,
    London.

Backer, T.E., Liberman, R.P. and Kuehnel, T.G. (1986) Dissemination and adoption of innovative psychosocial interventions, *Journal of Consulting and Clinical Psychology*, 54, 1, 111-118.

British Geriatrics Society (1994) *Guidelines for the Role of Community Geriatrician*, British Geriatrics Society, London.

Caldock, K. (1993) A preliminary study of changes in assessment: examining the relationship between recent policy and practitioners' knowledge, opinions and practice, *Health and Social Care in the Community*, 1, 3, 139-146.

Caldock, K. (1994) The new assessment: moving towards holism or new roads to fragmentation?, in D.J. Challis, B.P. Davies and K.J. Traske (eds) *Community Care: New Agendas and Challenges from the UK and Overseas*, Arena, Aldershot.

Challis, D.J. (1994) *Implementing Caring for People: Care Management: Factors Influencing its Development in the Implementation of Community Care*, Department of Health, London.

Challis, D.J., Darton, R.A., Johnson, L., Stone, M. and Traske, K.J. (1995) *Care Management and Health Care of Older People: The Darlington Community Care Project*, Arena, Aldershot.

Challis, D.J., Carpenter, I. and Traske, K.J. (1996) *Assessment in Continuing Care Homes: Towards a National Standard Instrument*, Personal Social Services Research Unit, University of Kent, Canterbury.

Challis, D.J., von Abendorff, R., Brown, P. and Chesterman, J.F. (1997) Care management and dementia: an evaluation of the Lewisham Intensive Case Management Scheme, in S. Hunter (ed.) *Research Highlights in Social Work 31. Dementia: Challenges and New Directions*, Jessica Kingsley Publishers, London.

Cm 849 (1989) *Caring for People: Community Care in the Next Decade and Beyond*, HMSO, London.

Dening, T. (1992) Community psychiatry of old age: a UK perspective, *International Journal of Geriatric Psychiatry*, 7, 10, 757-766.

Department of Health (1993) *Monitoring and Development: Assessment Special Study*, Department of Health, London.

Department of Health (1994) *Implementing Caring for People: Care Management*, Department of Health, London.

Fairweather, G.W., Sanders, D.H. and Tornatzky, L.G. with Harris, R.N. (1974) *Creating Change in Mental Health Organizations*, Pergamon, New York.

Ferlie, E.B., Challis, D.J. and Davies, B.P. (1989) *Efficiency-Improving Innovations in Social Care of the Elderly*, Gower, Aldershot.

Griffiths, R. (1988) *Community Care: Agenda for Action*, A Report to the Secretary of State for Social Services, HMSO, London.

Murphy, E. and Challis, D.J. (1993) The Lewisham Care Management Scheme for the Elderly, in World Health Organization, *Mental Health and Ageing*, World Health Organization, Geneva.

National Health Service and Community Care Act 1990 (1990 c. 19) HMSO, London.

2 Care Management and Community Care: Current Issues

Bob Welch

This chapter is intended to give a broad *tour d'horizon* of where the SSI feels it has reached with care management. At the time of writing it has been nearly five years since members of the SSI and others were involved in producing the original practice guidance: the Managers' and the Practitioners' Guides (SSI/SWSG, 1991a,b). It is, therefore, opportune to appraise how that guidance is being implemented. Managers and practitioners may remember that the SSI guidance hedged its bets by suggesting a range of models, within an overall framework, inviting experimentation, which, it is pleasing to say, has been done with relish! Managers, practitioners and the SSI have now together to take stock of what has been individually and corporately learnt from the very different and disparate experiences. The SSI is currently distilling a range of development issues from its inspection and monitoring work. These cover the whole gamut of care management arrangements, assessment procedures, interagency working, volume management, targeting, financial devolution, outcome measurement and the required skills for care management.

This chapter focuses on just four areas where, it appears, difficulty is being experienced:

- terminology;
- purchaser/provider separation;
- commissioning; and

• social work and care management.

Terminology

This section concentrates on five terms: care management, assessment of need, eligibility, objectives and targeting.

Care management

Despite everybody's best efforts, care management still appears to mean different things to different people. We are divided by a common language. That is why the SSI is seriously considering preparing its own glossary, spelling out, simply and briefly, what at least the SSI means by those terms, in the hope that it might prompt greater clarity in the ongoing debate about further implementation. The SSI said in the guidance that everyone in receipt of a continuing service should experience the process of care management. It did not say, despite contrary interpretations, that everyone should have a care manager throughout the process. The SSI did not know, when the guidance was written, how care management would pan out and which models would prove most appropriate. It appears that the pursuit of a holy grail, of one single model that is suited to all circumstances for all user groups, is being cancelled out. There may be a coherence of common principles, but, basically, the organisational structures have to grow out of what already exists and cannot be unilaterally imposed from on high. Therefore, some differentiation is inevitable and, in many cases, desirable. However, for any one user group, the SSI is coming to the view that there are probably four types of care management necessary to make up an integrated and comprehensive system, as shown in Table 2.1.

First, there is the administrative form that can be undertaken by receptioniststyle customer service officers. There has been a whole range of experimentation giving a higher status and profile to the initial information-processing at the point of reception, to initiate simple services. That is in addition to the enquiries that are dealt with without being translated into a specific referral. However, initiating simple services appears to represent only a small proportion of the work (5-10

Table 2.1. Differentiated approach

Skill	Needs	Assessment	Purpose of intervention	Proportion of referrals
Adminis-trative	Simple/ practical	Self/ single agency	Advice/ simple service	5-10%[a]
Vocational	Non-complex/ non-intensive/ stable	Limited/ one or two agencies	Support	60-70%[a]
Specialist	Limited/ intensive/ volatile	Specific/ one or two agencies	Rehabilitation	10-20%[a]
Professional	Complex/ intensive/ volatile	Comprehensive/ multi-agency	Support and/or rehabilitation	10-15%[a]

a Variable by user group.

per cent). The much greater volume of the referrals includes those that require a straightforward response to non-complex needs, for which many authorities are involving what they call care coordinators, described as the vocational form in Table 2.1. That, in the SSI's analysis, is the major bulk of the work (60-70 per cent). The third type is where only a specialist assessment and care plan is required for particular needs, such as rehabilitation (10-20 per cent). With hindsight, the SSI's guidance was mistaken in that it did not underline the crucial distinction that needs to be made between mainstream, ordinary care management and what the PSSRU used to call case management, which both now appear to call 'intensive care management' (Challis, 1994), the fourth category. This involves the designation of a care manager who combines the coordinating function with a therapeutic, supportive role for that minority of users who require such intensive involvement (10-15 per cent).

The trick of implementation would appear to be to ensure that the most qualified and expert personnel are targeted on the appropriate level of need. Logistically and financially, no authority can afford to spread that resource any more thinly than absolutely necessary. There are concerns that many care managers, however their responsibilities are defined, are being overwhelmed by the volume of work. Therefore, systems are breaking down; monitoring and review are sometimes not happening and sometimes falling by default to providers. Individual managers are developing survival strategies, but these have yet to be brought together into a coherent overall management strategy.

By and large, with few exceptions, most authorities have sought to build care management on the social work culture. There are a very few which have based it on the home help culture. Readers may wish to consider the implications of how they have oriented their own models in their own authorities. In the former, where there is emphasis on the intensive/therapeutic dimension, there tend to be increasing delays in the provision of simple services, whereas in the latter there is insufficient attention to the targeting of the intensive/ therapeutic dimension. There is a balance to be struck to ensure that all people with differing levels of need receive an efficient and effective service, and that available personnel are deployed to optimum effect.

In the last report on care management developments, published in August 1994 (Department of Health, 1994), some criteria for the allocation of care managers were suggested for the 'professional' variant of care management, as shown in Box 2.1.

To these three criteria, a fourth should be added, in terms of the scope to maximise health and social care gain. The test of a care manager is the value that they add to the process. The SSI is very concerned to promote a shift in focus from issues of process to an evaluation of outcomes, because, with ever tighter budgets, no-one can afford to

---

Box 2.1. Proposed criteria for allocation of a care manager

1. Where the needs and/or circumstances of the user are complex, high risk and/or volatile.

    or

2. Where the care plan is:
    a. volatile *or*
    b. requiring high status of coordination.

    or

3. Where a transfer of responsibility would jeopardise the user's acceptance of ongoing assistance or rehabilitation.

deploy personnel who are not adding value to the process. Of course, such care managers may also use their skills to contribute to the assessment of other users, besides their ongoing caseload, without subsequently having to remain involved.

Assessment of need

There is a real issue about the definition of need which cannot be addressed in the space available in this chapter, but about which much greater clarity and consensus is needed. However, there is also an issue about assessment. Some common understanding of what is meant by assessment is needed. It continues to be a concern that the scope of the assessment is over-expansive in many cases. There is an understandable professional imperative that drives people to ask more and more questions. To counter that imperative there would appear to be a need to define what is the least number of questions that must be asked in order to effect the necessary business. Proformas and procedures need to assist skilled personnel to exercise their discretion, to adjust the scope of the assessment to that necessary function. (Iain Carpenter discusses one approach to this later in the book.) There is still some way to go before the process is truly user-friendly and actually starts from where the user is and talks about what they want to talk about, rather than using checklists or ticking boxes! Unless great care is taken, these can get in the way of that crucial initial point of interaction between assessor and user.

It means starting from the difficulty or problem or whatever the user wants to call it, and taking that as the starting point of the assessment, accepting that a series of assessment interviews may be required, in response to successive referrals of particular needs: in other words, to proceed at the user's pace. It is bizarre to believe that people, who are total strangers, will open up their lives in one go, simply because the assessor is armed with a questionnaire that pries into every corner of their lives. They will want to test them out. If they can trust the assessor with a little bit of information, and the assessor then responds effectively, they may come back and disclose more and other deeper needs, but that trust has to be earned. It cannot be demanded as a bureaucratic right.

Having clarified the area of difficulty, it is necessary to establish what that user is motivated to do in relation to that difficulty and what they want to achieve. However, there should be a clear differentiation between the description of the needs, the user's aspirations in relation to those needs and the professional analysis or hypothesis as to the most appropriate way of responding to those needs. Everybody will have seen proformas which are endless descriptions of need, but nowhere do they effectively make such differentiations. Nor do they clearly sort out what are the difficulties that have causes which are the responsibility of other agencies, thereby validating the involvement of other agencies in the assessment process. Much more explicit and clear definitions of the scope and purpose of the assessment process are needed, not only for the assessor's own agency but also for other agencies, in order that a corporate diagnosis is available before decisions are made about eligibility for assistance. The community care reforms are all about accountable decision-making. Few assessment forms hold assessors to account in justifying their allocation of public resources against that agency's published eligibility criteria. It will be necessary to move to a much more explicit justification of decisions, as money gets ever tighter.

The final stage of assessment is the negotiation of an agreed objective or objectives of any intervention. It is a major area of disappointment in these early days of implementing care management that there does seem to have been a great difficulty in defining and recording objectives that have been agreed with users and carers, or even believing that such a process is necessary. The aim is to make that person's life better and not worse; and those objectives should be framed in ways that are measurable, so as to be able to hold providers to account for their achievement. That is a major professional challenge over the next few years.

In other words, what constitutes an assessment must be clearly defined, but, at the same time, without over-complicating the process. It is often possible to provide obvious and simple solutions to difficulties on the basis of limited assessment information. The emphasis must always be on what is the least, not the most, information required to provide an appropriate service.

Eligibility

There is confusion about different types and levels of eligibility, as to whether it refers to eligibility for assessment or for urgency or level of assessment, eligibility for resources or eligibility for individual services. Eligibility criteria are generally not yet framed in terms that are comprehensible to the general public or in terms that are owned and consistently applied by practitioners. In broad terms, the eligibility criteria that are currently being developed, at their root, focus on risk: risk to self, risk to or from others, risk to the support system or potential risk. As budgets are tightened, there is a tendency to concentrate on the higher levels of risk, focusing on the individual rather than the support system. The ideas which have come out of research work by Clare Wenger, on analysing support systems and their scope and capacity for providing different levels of care (Wenger, 1992), are very attractive, because this dimension is not currently given sufficient weight. However, the new Carers' Bill will encourage authorities to think more about indirect support options rather than leaping to direct support options, which may undermine informal care systems rather than complement and supplement them. At the same time as ensuring that available resources are deployed to maximum effect, it will be necessary to become more rigorous in focusing on those areas of risk where it is imperative and essential that the state intervenes because they cannot be managed in any other way by the individual, the family or the local community. These risk criteria have also to be translated across agency boundaries. Table 2.2 gives some indication of these cross-agency indicators of risk.

However, risk is only one dimension of eligibility; the other is that of health and social care gain. As in child care, there is growing recognition of the distinction between child protection and child support, so, in adult care, there is a necessary distinction between the inescapable interventions to manage identified risks and elective investment in users and carers where there is a projected health and/or social care gain. No authority can afford to be reduced to a merely reactive role in managing risk but needs to preserve a proactive role in promoting social well-being, albeit on a targeted, selective basis.

In that sense, decisions on intervention should ultimately be grounded in some form of cost-benefit analysis that spans all agencies and interest groups, deploying statutory resources, as illustrated in Table 2.3.

Table 2.2. Eligibility

Risk priority	Social services	Housing	Health
Risk to self	Self-neglect	Homeless/hazardous accommodation	Suicidal
Risk to others	Anti-social behaviour	Problem neighbours	Paranoid/ psychopathic
Risk from others	Adult abuse	Racial harassment	Neurotic
Risk to support system	Housework overload	Family overcrowding	Carer stress
Potential risk	Bereavement	Damp housing	Degenerative disease diagnosis

Table 2.3. Cost-benefit analysis format

Risk to			Potential gain to			Capital & revenue cost to	
User	Carers	Community	User	Carers	Community	Agency	Other agencies
Aggregate risk			Aggregate gain			Aggregate cost	

In such an analysis, acceptable cost parameters will obviously vary with the objective (see below) and the projected length of intervention. Where users and carers warrant different levels of priority, as between agencies, but where simultaneous investment would maximise the benefit, there needs to be some ring-fencing of resources in each agency to allow for allocations outside of the normal internal priority system. It is accepted that it may take some time to achieve this ideal.

Objectives

This is another difficult area to define. Some readers may feel that the following categorisation is somewhat medical in its orientation, but it is an attempt to reach across the health/social services divide towards common criteria of intervention:

- preventative;
- palliative;
- rehabilitative; and
- curative.

At the very least, it should challenge both health and social services authorities to consider whether they have investigated sufficiently the curative or rehabilitative options before settling for the merely palliative, which tends to be too often the case at present.

Targeting

Many authorities are now beginning to question this notion of focusing their resources increasingly on the most dependent, asking whether it is the most cost-effective way of deploying their resources. In other countries, and here also, in part, care management has been used as a means to effect what the PSSRU terms 'downward substitution': that is to say, moving people out of hospital and/or keeping them out of any institutional care, on the assumption that it not only accords better with people's wishes but that there are potential savings in resources. However, it has long been clear that, beyond a certain level of dependency, care at home involves levels of expenditure that have significant opportunity costs for other users. Authorities are increasingly addressing this issue by setting broad cost ceilings to care packages. At the very least, the hypothesis needs to be tested that there is more benefit to more people at less cost from low levels of investment in users in the initial stages of dependency (for example, two hours of home help per week), than in high-level investment in significantly fewer high-dependency users. Of course, these are not alternative options, but each authority has to strike its own balance.

Purchaser/provider separation

As was made plain in the Managers' and Practitioners' Guides to Care Management and Assessment (SSI/SWSG, 1991a,b), the SSI has never believed that a purist purchaser/provider separation was desirable or practicable. While it is essential for users' and carers' interests to be protected in the purchase of service, this does not mean that all care management responsibilities do or should fall to purchasers. In the last SSI report on care management (Department of Health, 1994) it was recognised that these responsibilities were increasingly being shared between purchasers and providers, but not always with the necessary safeguards in place because of the potential conflict of interest. These were listed as follows:

- managers/budget-holders of a particular service should not carry any care management responsibilities;
- purchasers and providers should ensure a separation in process between the assessment of need and care planning;
- monitoring and quality assurance systems should be established (for example, sampling by purchasers); and
- needs-led changes in care planning should not be constrained by a particular service or provider.

A prerequisite of such sharing is that both purchasers and providers receive the requisite training in care management skills. This provides a basis for partnership not only in assessment and care planning but also in monitoring and review. The actual distribution of responsibilities will vary according to the complexity of need and the number of services involved. The imperative is to distribute them in a pragmatic way with adequate safeguards, so as to drive down transaction costs, while ensuring that the actual distribution of responsibilities is clearly understood by all concerned.

Commissioning

This is a new concept that is not yet fully understood. It refers to the purchasing of services within a strategic framework. Care management can only be truly needs-led if it is backed up by a commissioning process that is similarly needs-led. This is still rarely the case, in that services continue to be commissioned on an historical basis without reference to changing patterns of need or user and carer choice. This is because population needs assessment is still at an embryonic stage and there is still not, in most authorities, systematic feedback to the commissioning process from individual assessments of need.

The practice guidance on care management encouraged the progressive devolution of commissioning responsibility, but only when the necessary financial management systems were in place. In the absence of such systems, some authorities have experienced difficulties and quickly retracted commissioning responsibility back to the centre. Yet other authorities have devolved commissioning responsibility without any clarity or interagency agreement on which services are most appropriately commissioned at what level in the organisation: for example, commissioning the most specialist minority services at the highest levels of aggregation.

Clarity about commissioning responsibility becomes all the more important where it may vary between services and between agencies. That is why the Department has recently issued further guidance on joint commissioning, to be followed up by a workbook to assist health and local authorities to both clarify and develop their commissioning arrangements. In the NHS, commissioning responsibility is being devolved to variants of GP fundholding, so there is increasing scope to progress joint or complementary commissioning at locality level. That, in turn, opens up opportunities to involve the public in commissioning decisions in a more meaningful way, as will, more specifically, the proposal to give direct payments to purchase their own services.

Because these commissioning arrangements will vary so markedly between localities that will not always have interagency coterminosity, it is essential that practitioners are kept up to date with these rapidly evolving options for commissioning, not least because many practitioners retain an ambivalence about assuming a commissioning role at all. Some prefer to act as advocates for users, negotiating with first-line managers who hold the budgets. However, micro- and macro-purchasing are only ever likely to be effectively integrated, to the advantage of users and carers, where managers and practitioners share the commissioning responsibility, recognising the opportunity costs to other users and potential users of the resource allocation to any one user, even if that means that the advocacy role has to pass increasingly to independent agencies.

Social work and care management

It would be inappropriate for social work to seek to resolve its identity crisis by colonising care management. The practice guidance on care management recognised the particular relevance of social work skills to care management but, equally, made clear that practitioners from any of the caring professions could undertake care management or coordinating responsibilities. There is a case for saying that social work, just like all the other care disciplines, should have a therapeutic value in its own right, to warrant being purchased. For that very reason, a few social services authorities have established social work provider units, acknowledging that, in recent years, there has perhaps been an over-emphasis on the provision of practical services to the neglect of emotional and psychological problems, with a consequent withering of counselling and therapeutic skills. How many elderly people are being admitted to residential or nursing homes who are in fact depressed, and in need of counselling rather than any relocation that may ultimately compound their depression?

As argued elsewhere in this chapter, most social services referrals require the practical skills of coordination on a continuing basis. This is not to deny that some of those referrals might benefit from time-limited social work intervention of a therapeutic kind. However, social work skills may be most appropriate for that minority of users for whom services need to be coordinated within the context of an ongoing supportive relationship with a care manager. This suggests that social services authorities should perhaps review their current skill mixes and use social workers in more selective and targeted ways, allied to greater use of more vocationally-trained personnel.

Such considerations acquire some urgency as the NHS shifts its priority from acute to primary care with the introduction of GP fundholding and a range of supporting multidisciplinary community-based teams. This brings into question the whole deployment of health and social services personnel and their distribution across primary care, specialist community-based care and secondary care. There is clearly a need for better communication and coordination between health and social services at the primary care level. However, it is not clear whether this is best accomplished through outposting social workers to GP surgeries, or through vocationally-trained coordinators who deal with the majority of social services needs themselves but refer those with more intensive, specialist needs to multidisciplinary teams in which social workers are full members.

What is now needed is a lively period of experimentation at the health, social services and, possibly, housing interface, in which the performance of different combinations of staff, with differently defined competencies, will be carefully evaluated to establish which make the most cost-effective impact on health and social care need.

Future development of care management

When the Department of Health has completed its internal review of what has been learnt so far about the implementation of care management, the SSI will need to consider whether any further guidance of a generic nature is required or what other stimulus can be given to the ongoing development of care management.

However, the SSI believes that care management needs to be differentially developed to suit different user group needs and different levels of need, as well as local organisational circumstances. The test of effectiveness should increasingly be the outcomes that these different arrangements are able to achieve for users and carers. For that reason, the Department of Health is actively considering the commissioning of surveys of research, on a user group basis, looking at which interventions and which ways of delivering those interventions are most effective, in effect copying similar work in the child care field. The Department would want to disseminate what is known widely to the field and, by identifying the current gaps in knowledge, establish priorities for future research.

Over the first two years of implementation, everybody has been on a steep learning curve about care management. There has been a wide range of experimental approaches, but what has been learnt has yet to be consolidated; still less has been achieved, on a generalised basis, in that essential shift in culture from a service-led to a needs-led approach.

Indeed, with ever-tightening budgets, there is a danger that the pursuit of a genuinely needs-led approach will be abandoned and social services authorities will relapse back to their traditional ways. That must not be allowed to happen. Care management is no panacea, but, sensibly and pragmatically applied, it does provide a process for allocating available resources to meet needs in a more creative and cost-effective way.

References

Challis, D.J. (1994) *Implementing Caring for People: Care Management: Factors Influencing its Development in the Implementation of Community Care*, Department of Health, London.

Department of Health (1994) *Implementing Caring for People: Care Management*, Department of Health, London.

Social Services Inspectorate and Social Work Services Group (SSI/SWSG) (1991a) *Care Management and Assessment: Managers' Guide*, HMSO, London.

Social Services Inspectorate and Social Work Services Group (SSI/SWSG) (1991b) *Care Management and Assessment: Practitioners' Guide*, HMSO, London.

Wenger, G.C. (1992) *Help in Old Age – Facing up to Change: A Longitudinal Network Study*, Liverpool University Press, Liverpool.

3 Community Care and Health Care for Older People

Jackie Morris

Demand for health and social care

The number of older people in the population in the United Kingdom has greatly increased this century, with a rapid acceleration over the last two decades. The total population is projected to continue to increase for the next 30 years or so, rising to about 62.2 million in 2026 (Office of Population Censuses and Surveys, 1993), after which deaths will exceed births. Over the next 40 years the proportion aged 45 and over is projected to rise from 37 per cent in 1991 to nearly 50 per cent in 2061. It is thought that the number of persons aged over 75 could double by the middle of the next century. But over the next few years, to the end of the decade, although the number of young and old people will decline slightly, the numbers of very old people will increase by 30 per cent. There are now 400,000 more people aged 85 and over than there were twenty years ago. By the year 2000 there will be approximately 1.1 million people aged over 85, 250,000 more people of this age than in 1991 in England.

Over the last 150 years the average life expectancy at birth has risen from 40 years to over 70 years. The average life expectancy for men is now 73 years and that for women is 79 years. Ageing is associated with an increased perception of poor health, and disability itself increases with age. Pessimists have argued that an ageing population will be accompanied by a pandemic of degenerative diseases and chronic mental disorders. Optimists believe that the adoption of healthier life-styles will result in a compression of morbidity into an increasingly brief period before death. Others are of the opinion that in reality there will be a firm balance between the two (Robine and Ritchie, 1991).

An understanding of the 1980 World Health Organization classification of the consequences of impairments, disabilities and handicaps is essential when planning services for older people. It helps to explain the relationship between health and social care. Disease or pathology refers to the damage and abnormal processes occurring within an organ. Impairments are any loss or abnormality of physical, psychological or anatomical function and tend to be the doctor's principal concern. Disability is the loss of an ability to carry out an essential activity of daily living as a consequence of an impairment. Handicaps are the social consequence of pathology or disease and can be expressed as the disadvantage suffered by the individual as the result of their disability (World Health Organization, 1980).

An example could be an individual who has suffered a stroke (disease). They are therefore no longer able to move an arm or leg (impairment), and are therefore no longer able to dress themselves or walk (disability). Their handicap will be that they will no longer be able to live by themselves without outside help.

The Department of Health has recently commissioned work (Bone et al., 1995) on Disability Free Life Expectancy, a measure of health and morbidity (disability) as a proportion of life expectancy. In addition to the finding that there appears to have been a national increase in incidence of medium levels of disability, there is a suggestion that the incidence of severe disability has decreased. The evidence from this work and the results of the General Household Survey also show that, from a population perspective, women spend a greater proportion of their life with disability than men. More older women than men report problems with simple activities of daily living. In the population aged over 75, nearly 20 per cent of women and 10 per cent of men cannot cut their own toenails; 10 per cent of men and nearly 30 per cent of women cannot walk outside; and approximately 20 per cent of women and 10 per cent of men cannot bath themselves (Bone et al., 1995). Cognitive impairment/dementia occurs in up to 20 per cent of people aged over 80 (Hofman et al., 1991). Higher levels of both physical disability (dependency) and dementia have been found in both the residential and the nursing home sector (Department of Health, 1992; Bone et al., 1995).

Not only have the numbers of older people increased, but the lifestyles of older people have also changed over the last few years. Women now form 57 per cent of the population aged over 60, and 65 per cent of those over 75. Whereas in the past many older people lived in shared accommodation, now nearly 50 per cent of older women and 20 per cent of older men live alone. Seventy-six per cent of older men and 46 per cent of older women are married. Divorce is far more common than it was twenty years ago, and the proportion of women aged between 45-54 who work has increased from 62 per cent in 1971 to an expected 77 per cent in 2001. Activities decline with age; the most popular leisure activity is watching television. Twenty-seven per cent of people aged over 60 smoked, of whom 30 per cent were smoking twenty or more cigarettes per day. The number of older people taking regular exercise is small (Askham et al., 1992).

Although the ratio of older women to older men is expected to decrease during the next twenty years (Office of Population Censuses and Surveys, 1993), the proportion of older people living alone is expected to increase because of the increasing divorce rate, and other changes in family life. Changes in future patterns of care will also be affected by the overall level of employment, shifts in employment patterns, changes in productivity, and immigration, as well as the availability of those with appropriate skills. The socio-economic status of older people will influence their health status as well as their ability to continue to live in their own homes.

Service system change

The last ten years have seen a tremendous shift in the delivery of care, from hospital to the community. Traditionally, in the 1960s and 1970s, the frail old were cared for in NHS long-stay institutions and local authority-run residential homes. However, the increased use of income support to buy nursing or residential care in the independent sector dramatically changed the balance of care during the 1980s. The number of older people living in this sector has doubled over the last ten to fifteen years, and the social security budget for it has risen from £10 million in 1979 to £2.5 billion in 1992. In 1992 local authorities provided approximately 104,000 residential places, whereas they provided 137,000 places in the mid-1980s. The number of NHS long-stay beds decreased from 75,000 in 1970, to 65,000 in 1990. There are thought to be about 1.7 million people heavily involved in hands-on care, and the cost of unpaid care has been estimated at about £33.9 billion pounds (Nuttall et al., 1994).

Hospital services for older people have moved from their base in separate hospitals or isolated sanatoria or asylums, to acute hospitals where older people can have access to all the facilities of a modern hospital. No longer is there such a problem recruiting good nursing and medical personnel to work in wards or hospitals caring for older people.

The capacity to respond to treatment is the same in the old and the young. Hospital services have evolved to ensure that the acutely ill older person has immediate access to investigation and treatment by appropriately trained medical and nursing staff (Royal College of Physicians, 1994). In addition, the importance of rehabilitation, enabling them to cope with their disabilities and to achieve their optimal levels of physical, psychological and physiological function (by reducing handicap) has also been widely recognised (Stuck et al., 1993). The hospital admission rate for older people has increased considerably; this has been attributed to advances in medical treatment as well as greater expectations among individual older people. The average length of stay for patients in geriatric medicine has been dramatically reduced over the last twenty years, to a median figure of twelve days in 1992-93, although elderly people admitted with acute problems stay in hospital for even shorter periods (Department of Health, 1995a).

Recent developments have included hospital discharge schemes and 'hospital at home' to enable older people to return home more quickly after major illnesses, and the Darlington study has encouraged the development of care management schemes. The acute facilities in hospital are often supplemented by day hospital services offering rehabilitation and treatment without admission. There are now over 500 consultants in geriatric medicine, and most run a mixture of acute, rehabilitation and long-stay facilities. All services work as multidisciplinary teams and have developed tremendous expertise in the special problems faced by older people.

The psychiatry of old age has undergone a similar metamorphosis over the last 30 years. Starting with a handful of consultants in the 1960s, there are now about 250 consultants who provide a comprehensive service for older people with mental health problems. They too have moved away from an asylum-based practice to a preventive and rehabilitative approach. Old age psychiatrists also work in multidisciplinary teams and usually assess people in their own homes.

The nature of health problems in old age

Older people's medical problems are different, difficult and require expertise; they tend to suffer from multiple pathology and may have an atypical presentation of disease, and often have a combination of psychiatric and physical disease. They may take a longer time to recover from their acute illnesses, and often develop mobility problems as well as urinary and/or faecal incontinence when ill.

The most important cause of hospital admission, GP attendances, disability and death is cardiovascular disease, giving rise to coronary heart disease and stroke. The incidence of stroke (first-ever events) rises exponentially with age. Fifty per cent of strokes occur in people aged over 75. In a population of 250,000 there are approximately 3,000 stroke patients at one time, of whom half are severely disabled. After six months, 25 per cent of all stroke patients will be dead and 25 per cent will be dependent (disabled). The last twenty years have seen a drop in mortality from stroke, despite a rise in the numbers of people admitted to hospital. There is conclusive evidence showing that multidisciplinary stroke rehabilitation in hospital reduces mortality and also improves outcome (Kalra et al., 1993; Sandercock, 1993). The next twenty years may see similar reductions in mortality, but the numbers of older people with disability arising from stroke will probably continue to rise as the population ages.

There is also a progressive increase in both the attack rate and the case fatality of myocardial infarction (heart attack) with increasing age. There is a 19 per cent prevalence rate of angina for people aged over 65. Coronary heart disease is the commonest cause of cardiac failure and death in older people, and is associated with reduced ability to carry out a range of activities, depending on severity, from dressing and getting out of bed, to being able to walk to the shops; even more dramatic strides have been made in its treatment than in that of stroke. Older people have been found to respond as well as younger people to modern therapeutic intervention such as thrombolytic therapy (clot busters) (Elder and Fox, 1992).

The other major cause of longstanding illness giving rise to disability in old age is osteoarthritis. Osteoarthritis causes chronic pain and disability. The main joints affected are the hip and the knee. Surveys show that self-reported joint pain, arthritis and observed locomotor disability are strongly age-related. Hip osteoarthritis has a roughly equal sex incidence, and its prevalence gradually increases with age. Fifty per cent of those aged over 65 are significantly affected by osteoarthritis. Drugs for this condition are not only expensive but are also responsible for many unpleasant side-effects in older patients. A large proportion of the personal social services' bill is spent on people with disability secondary to osteoarthritis. It has been estimated that 2.5 per cent of all community health and social care is provided to people whose primary diagnosis is osteoarthritis. Pain and the consequent disability are the main symptoms. Pain management can often be unsuccessful, but simple measures such as activity, proper footwear and physiotherapy can greatly improve the patient's outcome. Research is in progress to further evaluate effective treatments (Medical Research Council, 1994).

There are thought to be approximately 600,000 people with dementia in England. A health district of 250,000 will have at least 3,000 people aged over 60 with the condition, of whom one-third will be severely affected. People with a mild form of the disease may just be forgetful and this can easily be mistaken for normal ageing. People in the advanced stages of the disease may be unable to undertake simple activities of daily living: for example, washing, eating and dressing. Sufferers can be disorientated in time and space, developing incontinence of urine and faeces, as well as behavioural problems and, eventually, in the terminal stages, require help with all activities of daily living. The commonest causes of dementia are Alzheimer's disease and multiple strokes. At present there is no specific treatment available, but effective organisation and coordination of care can improve the quality of life of both the patient and the carer. At present, 13 per cent of elderly people with this disease live alone, 37 per cent live in institutions and half live with carers (Morris, 1993).

Depression is also common, and is underdiagnosed and undertreated in old age. Studies have shown prevalence rates ranging between 11 and 19.5 per cent. Depression rates are higher, estimated at about 38 per cent, in residential care. Twenty-nine per cent of older medical admissions are thought to show significant depressive features, of whom 9 per cent show evidence of severe depression. Despite evidence to show that older people benefit from treatment as much as younger people, only a small minority actually are treated. For many, age does not affect prognosis (Walker and Katona, 1995).

Accidents are also an important cause of ill health and death in this age group. Over 300,000 people aged 65 and over attend accident and emergency units, having fallen. Of these, 59 per cent of falls occur within the home, and individuals falling at home are more frail and have a worse prognosis than those who fall while walking outside. Seventy per cent of all fatal home accidents occur in people aged 65 and over. Hip fractures are the commonest major sequelae of a fall. Hip fracture rates have doubled over the last twenty years to about 55,000 cases in 1989 (Morris, 1994). They too are associated with significant mortality and disability, but targeted rehabilitation in hospital also shortens length of hospital stay and improves outcome (Currie, 1994).

Other causes of ill health in old age are respiratory disease, osteoporosis and cancer. Less common, but a major cause of illness in this age group, is Parkinson's disease. Problems with eyesight and hearing increase with age and are often badly managed.

Towards more integrated care

Primary, secondary and tertiary prevention of disease is an effective approach for managing disease and disability, both in the hospital and the community setting. Primary prevention or health promotion is the prevention of disease: for example, by the use of 'flu vaccination or by the introduction of exercise classes in sheltered accommodation to improve physical function. Secondary prevention is the treatment of asymptomatic disease leading to the development of severe disease; for example, the treatment of hypertension in older people has been proven to be effective in the reduction of incidence of fatal strokes (Medical Research Council Working Party, 1992). Tertiary prevention is the treatment of the disease itself, thereby reducing disability (for example, stroke rehabilitation). Ways of introducing this in the community should be developed and evaluated in order to inform purchasers and providers of care.

The wholesale transfer of care of frail older people from the hospital setting to that of the community has shifted the medical responsibility from the hospital consultants and their teams to the general practitioner. General practitioners are being asked to care for an increasingly sick and disabled population, without any shift of resources. Only about 30 per cent of general practitioners have training in geriatric medicine and far fewer in old age psychiatry. There is also increasing evidence that the current yearly 75+ check (completed by GPs on patients at and above this age) has been poorly implemented, is not popular with GPs and does not work. In many cases treatable disease remains unidentified until it is untreatable and irreversible (Williams and Wallace, 1993).

Many other developed countries have experienced very similar shifts in care: for example, in Australia the Aged Care Reforms introduced mandatory assessments through specially-designed Geriatric Assessment Teams to ensure that older people were appropriately placed. Increased resources were introduced through a system of case management and improved coordinated home care resulting in a reduction in the use of the residential and nursing home sector (Quartararo and O'Neill, 1990).

The implementation of *Caring for People* (Cm 849, 1989) made local authorities responsible for funding those seeking public support in private and voluntary homes, for assessing individual needs, and for designing care arrangements and securing their delivery within available resources. The budget for social care, both in the domiciliary and the residential sector, was transferred from social security to local authorities. It was intended that the legislation would encourage health and social service purchasers and providers to work more closely together. Sadly, care for older people is becoming increasingly fragmented and inadequate, and the lessons of Darlington have not been applied nationally. Assessments of need by the social worker are not always done in concert with doctors and therapists. There has been a failure, on the whole, to understand the importance of regular multidisciplinary review and monitoring, with a view to further rehabilitation when necessary.

While health care is free at the point of delivery and social care is means-tested, the planning of joint services is fraught with difficulties. Nowhere is this more difficult than in the care of frail older people who were traditionally the responsibility of the health service.

The success of community care depends on collaboration between health and social services to ensure that older people receive the right balance of care. The importance of close multidisciplinary working and the need for skilled social workers in this area have been recognised by the Department of Health (1994, 1995b). One method of planning and developing services would be to bring together, in a more systematic fashion, information from the 75+ GP checks with the social workers' needs assessments, facilitating purchasers to buy services to meet both population and individual needs.

In order to deliver care in the community, multidisciplinary teams with specialist expertise will need to be developed and evaluated, to work alongside general practitioners, in collaboration with social services. In addition, specialist teams will need to work in the residential and nursing home sector, to enable their staff to keep up to date with advances in the management of older people, thus ensuring that residents receive prompt appropriate treatment, as well as setting standards of care which can be monitored. This service should be available to older people whether they are in the state or the private and voluntary sectors.

The future scenario for older people could be very exciting. It is doubtful whether the situation will continue as now, and they could become a much more powerful and vocal group, no longer prepared to put up with second-rate services in the community. High technology in the home and the hospital could enable radical new developments to take place allowing older people, and their carers, to have far greater freedoms than previously imagined.

References

Askham, J., Barry, C., Grundy, E., Hancock, R. and Tinker, A. (1992) *Life After 60*, Age Concern Institute of Gerontology, King's College London.

Bone, M.R., Bebbington, A.C., Jagger, C., Morgan, K. and Nicholaas, G. (1995) *Health Expectancy and Its Uses*, HMSO, London.

Cm 849 (1989) *Caring for People: Community Care in the Next Decade and Beyond*, HMSO, London.

Currie, C.T. (1994) Early supported discharge for elderly trauma patients: a report on a preliminary study, *Clinical Rehabilitation*, 8, 207-12.

Department of Health (1992) *The Health of Elderly People. An Epidemiological Overview: Companion Papers*, Central Health Monitoring Unit Epidemiological Overview Series, Companion Papers to Volume 1, HMSO, London.

Department of Health (1994) *Hospital Discharge Workbook: A Manual on Hospital Discharge Practice*, Department of Health, London.

Department of Health (1995a) *Hospital Episode Statistics. Volume 1. Finished Consultant Episodes by Diagnosis, Operation and Specialty. England: Financial Year 1992-93*, Department of Health, London.

Department of Health (1995b) *NHS Responsibilities for Meeting Continuing Health Care Needs*, HSG(95)8, LAC(95)5, Department of Health, London.

Elder, A.T. and Fox, K.A.A. (1992) Thrombolytic treatment for elderly patients, *British Medical Journal*, 305, 846-7.

Hofman, A., Rocca, W.A., Brayne, C., Breteler, M.M.B., Clarke, M., Cooper, B., Copeland, J.R.M., Dartigues, J.F., Da Silva Droux, A., Hagnell, O., Heeren, T.J., Engedal, K., Jonker, C., Lindesay, J., Lobo, A., Mann, A.H., Mölsä, P.K., Morgan, K., O'Connor, D.W., Sulkava, R., Kay, D.W.K. and Amaducci, L. (1991) The prevalence of dementia in Europe: a collaborative study of 1980-1990 findings, *International Journal of Epidemiology*, 20, 736-48.

Kalra, L., Dale, P. and Crome, P. (1993) Improving stroke rehabilitation, a controlled study, *Stroke*, 24, 1462-7.

Medical Research Council (1994) *The Health of the UK's Elderly People*, Medical Research Council, London.

Medical Research Council Working Party (1992) Medical Research Council trial of treatment of hypertension: principal results, *British Medical Journal*, 304, 405-12.

Morris, J. (1993) Dementia: caring for the carers, *Health Trends*, 25, 1, 3.

Morris, J. (1994) Falls in older people, Editorial, *Journal of the Royal Society of Medicine*, 87, 435-6.

Nuttall, S.R., Blackwood, R.J.L., Bussell, B.M.H., Cliff, J.P., Cornall, M.J., Cowley, A., Gatenby, P.L. and Webber, J.M. (1994) Financing long-term care in Great Britain, *Journal of the Institute of Actuaries*, 121, 1, 1-68.

Office of Population Censuses and Surveys (1993) *National Population Projections 1991-based. Report and Microfiche giving Population Projections by Sex and Age for the United Kingdom, Great Britain and Constituent Countries*, Series PP2 no. 18, HMSO, London.

Quartararo, M. and O'Neill, T.J. (1990) Nursing home admissions: the effect of a multidisciplinary assessment team on the frequency of admission approvals, *Community Health Studies*, 14, 441-9.

Robine, J.M. and Ritchie, K. (1991) Healthy life expectancy: evaluation of global indicator of change in population health, *British Medical Journal*, 302, 457-60.

Royal College of Physicians (1994) *Ensuring Equity and Quality of Care for Elderly People. The Interface between Geriatric Medicine and General (Internal) Medicine*, Royal College of Physicians of London, London.

Sandercock, P. (1993) Managing stroke: the way forward, *British Medical Journal*, 307, 1297-8.

Stuck, A.E., Siu, A.L., Wieland, G.D., Adams, J. and Rubenstein, L.Z. (1993) Comprehensive geriatric assessment: a meta-analysis of controlled trials, *The Lancet*, 342, 1032-6.

Walker, Z. and Katona, C.L.E. (1995) Depression in elderly people with physical illness, *Current Medical Literature: Geriatrics*, 8, 1, 3-7.

Williams, E.I. and Wallace, P. (1993) *Health Checks for People Aged 75 and Over*, Occasional Paper 59, Royal College of General Practitioners, London.

World Health Organization (1980) *International Classification of Impairments, Disabilities and Handicaps: A Manual of Classification Relating to the Consequences of Disease*, World Health Organization, Geneva.

4 The Darlington Study: Findings and Lessons for Care Management, Health Care and Community Care

David Challis, Robin Darton and Karen Stewart

This chapter has two aims. First, to summarise some of the key findings from the Darlington study in order to set the context for the rest of this book. Second, to identify some of the potential areas of development for the future of community care that are offered by these findings and this approach to care management. Thus, it links with the themes developed in the other chapters of this book. The relevance of this study is the way in which it highlights the importance of refocusing aspects of assessment and care management for the future development of community care and its relationship with health.

The Darlington study

This study is one of a family of studies which have been undertaken by the PSSRU, over some years. These studies have looked at how the care management approach can work in different settings for vulnerable elderly people. The settings have been in social care within social services, within linked social care and primary care settings, and secondary care settings, such as geriatric services and psychogeriatric services. These studies have been targeted upon elderly people at high risk of entry to institutional care. The Darlington study built on the care management models developed in Kent and Gateshead (Challis and Davies,

1986; Davies and Challis, 1986; Challis et al., 1988, 1990, 1993), and extended these into a joint health and social services model of provision, based upon a geriatric multidisciplinary team (Challis et al., 1991a,b, 1995).

The origins of the Darlington Project began back in the 1980s when the Department of Health was trying to pump-prime new initiatives in community-based care. It was one of 28 pilot projects centrally funded under the government's Care in the Community Initiative (DHSS, 1983), and was designed to offer alternatives to long-stay care for physically frail elderly people. The initial focus was on existing inpatients, as had originally been planned: that is, patients who were located in long-stay hospital care. Increasingly, however, and entirely sensibly and realistically, the focus subsequently shifted to pre-placement decision-making processes, when individuals had been assessed as requiring long-stay hospital care. With the ending of central government funding, the project was incorporated, in a modified form, into the community unit of the district health authority.

The project team was employed by the social services department, and consisted of a project manager, three service managers whose role was to act as care managers, and a team of home care assistants. The care managers had to cost the service they provided to clients, working to an average budget of two-thirds of the cost of a long-stay hospital bed. The care managers were members of the geriatric multidisciplinary team, through which all referrals were directed. Thus the model of care which was developed linked secondary health care provision, that is a geriatric service, with a social care intervention involving care management. The service model is shown in Figure 4.1, and indicates the relationship between the project team and other professional staff, and the activities which were undertaken with the home care assistants, and with elderly people and their carers. The project team and other professional staff worked both directly with elderly people and their carers, and indirectly through the home care assistants. The broken line in Figure 4.1 indicates the feedback from clients, carers and home care assistants.

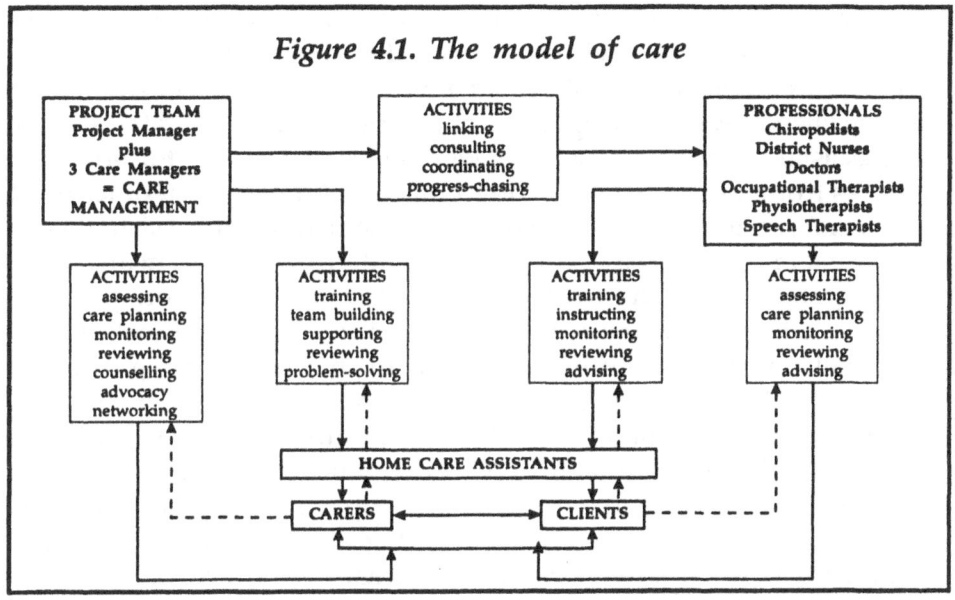

Figure 4.1. The model of care

The service in practice

One hundred and one elderly people were discharged from hospital to the project. Their average age was 80 years, and two-thirds were female. Over 90 per cent had been in hospital for two years or under. The most common cause of impairment was stroke, which afflicted over one-third of the elderly people. Most had severe mobility and self-care problems, and about two-thirds experienced problems in maintaining continence. Depression or anxiety appeared to be evident in the majority of the group, and nearly one-third suffered from confusional states. On the basis of the Behaviour Rating Scale from the Clifton Assessment Procedures for the Elderly (Pattie and Gilleard, 1979), the project clients were similar to patients in an acute medical ward.

Those elderly people who were to receive the service were assessed by the geriatric multidisciplinary team, comprising medical staff, hospital and community nursing staff, social workers, paramedical staff and the care managers from the project. The care managers coordinated the assessments of the elderly persons from the different professionals in the multidisciplinary team, and took responsibility for assessing the family and the potential support network. In about half the cases a home visit was undertaken with the elderly person, so that the suitability of the person's home environment could be assessed.

Each care manager was allocated a budget for their caseload of about twenty clients. A large proportion of this budget was allocated to home care assistant time, but resources were also used to pay for additional services from members of the community, and the input of other health and social services resources was also costed. Home care assistants were instructed and used by a variety of different professionals, in an attempt to integrate much of the work of several different 'hands-on' providers into the activities of one single care worker. Thus the functions of a home help, an auxiliary nurse or an aide to an occupational group were combined in one person. This was aimed at reducing the overlap and duplication of tasks and to provide more coordinated care to individual elderly people. The care managers' prime function was, in consultation with the multidisciplinary team, to develop, coordinate and regularly review a package of care, linking together all the necessary resources from a range of different providers, formal and informal. As well as the tasks of monitoring, liaison and coordination, this role also required the care manager to give considerable amounts of emotional support and advice to the elderly people and their families, complementing the activities of informal carers, and to provide support to the home care assistants and resolve conflicts in the care network.

Outcomes

The study compared individuals receiving services from the project with a similar group of patients identified in long-stay wards of an adjacent health district, which was seen as providing a reasonably similar style of geriatric service. The informal carers of both groups were also interviewed, focusing on the experience of care and degree of burden, and were also compared with a third group of carers of elderly people who were receiving the usual range of health and social services while living in the community.

Table 4.1 indicates the location of the elderly people in the project and the comparison group at six and twelve months after initial interviews. About two-thirds of the project group were still in their own homes after six months and only three people were in institutional care;

Table 4.1. Destinational outcomes at six and twelve months

Location	Project group		Comparison group	
	6 months	12 months	6 months	12 months
	%	%	%	%
At home	66	56	12	9
Institutional care	3	4	78	60
Dead	31	40	11	31
Number of cases	101	101	113	113

Overall chi-squared tests: at 6 months X^2 = 123.96 (p<0.001); at 12 months X^2 = 89.80 (p<0.001).

the remainder had died during the period. After twelve months, over 50 per cent were still at home. Although there was a significantly higher death rate in the project group after six months, this was not evident at twelve months, after allowing for the higher proportion of project clients (fifteen compared with one) who were terminally ill. Excluding the elderly people who were terminally ill, 30 per cent of both groups had died by twelve months. Over the first six months (182 possible days), project clients were at home for an average of 137 days, and the number of days in any form of institutional care was very small.

The outcomes of the project for the elderly people were measured by examining the differences between interview data collected before hospital discharge and six months after discharge, and equivalent measures were derived for the comparison group. Table 4.2 shows the mean change scores for subjective wellbeing, behavioural indicators, and quality of care indicators. For indicators of subjective wellbeing there was a statistically significant improvement in overall morale, a nearly statistically significant improvement in a measure of satisfaction with their current life situation, and a greater reduction in depression for those elderly people receiving the project compared with the comparison group. The project group also experienced a very significant reduction in loneliness. On most of the behavioural indicators derived from the CAPE BRS (Pattie and Gilleard, 1979) there were, unsurprisingly, no significant changes over time. However, those elderly people receiving the project did experience a significant reduction in apathy, compared with those remaining in hospital. This could be

Table 4.2. Client wellbeing: mean change scores over six months

	Project group	Comparison group	p value[a]
Subjective wellbeing			
General satisfaction	0.79	0.08	0.056
Satisfaction with life development	0.18	0.10	ns
Morale	1.74	0.21	0.037
Depression	-2.88	-1.05	<0.01
Loneliness	-0.84	0.23	<0.001
Number of cases (minimum)[b]	38	72	
Behavioural indicators (CAPE BRS)			
Physical disability	0.19	0.17	ns
Apathy	-0.62	0.12	0.014
Communication difficulties	0.07	0.11	ns
Social disturbance	0.60	0.09	ns
BRS total score	0.33	0.56	ns
Number of cases (minimum)[b]	66	99	
Quality of care indicators			
Need for improvement in level of care	-4.94	-0.22	<0.001
Social activity level	6.48	2.08	0.011
Number of cases (minimum)[b]	42	76	

a F-test. 'ns' = not significant.
b Minimum number of cases for which a comparison could be made, due to variable
non-response to individual questions, losses due to deaths and missing initial data
for project clients who entered the project at the beginning.

accounted for by the greater control they had gained over their lives
since their discharge from hospital, and an increase in their level of
social activity, which is also shown in Table 4.2. A more practical
indicator, that of quality of care, reveals that the project clients experienced a significantly reduced need for additional care, indicating a
marked reduction in the shortfall between need and what was actually
provided for them by the service.

Overall, it appears that those elderly people who were discharged
to the project were better off by most criteria than comparison group
patients remaining in long-stay hospital care. Few spent time in other

forms of care. Despite a higher death rate at six months, project clients also experienced significantly greater wellbeing in terms of their quality of life, significantly greater social activity and better quality of care, compared with the comparison group.

Carers of project clients were compared with two other groups: carers of elderly people in long-stay hospital care who were part of the client comparison group; and carers of elderly people who attended the day hospital in Darlington, but otherwise received traditional support at home. Table 4.3 shows summary indicators, as mean scores, of tasks performed and behaviours and burdens experienced, the carers' subjective feelings of distress associated with these (Platt et al., 1983; Platt, 1985) and, finally, the levels of malaise or stress experienced (Rutter et al., 1970). Project carers undertook fewer care tasks than day hospital

Table 4.3. Carer behavioural, burden and stress indicators: mean scores

	Project	Hospital	Day hospital	p value[a]	Significant group differences[b]
Behavioural and burden indicators[c]					
Care tasks undertaken	6.7	na	7.9	<0.05	na
Elderly person's behaviour	13.6	14.8	18.4	ns	–
Burdens experienced	4.4	5.3	6.3	<0.05	–
Number of cases (minimum)	63	25	28		
Subjective indicators[c]					
Distress — care tasks	4.7	na	9.8	<0.01	na
Distress — behaviour	12.9	17.6	24.1	<0.001	§, †
Distress — burdens	4.5	5.6	7.3	<0.05	§
Malaise score[d]	6.1	8.9	7.2	<0.05	‡
Number of cases (minimum)	62	27	26		

'na' = not applicable.
a Analysis of variance. 'ns' = not significant.
b Key to paired comparisons (Newman-Keuls test):
   § Project v Day hospital significant at 0.05 level.
   † Day hospital v Hospital significant at 0.05 level.
   ‡ Project v Hospital significant at 0.05 level.
c Platt (1985).
d Rutter et al. (1970).

carers, and experienced significantly less distress associated with this. While all three groups faced similar levels of behaviour problems, the day hospital carers were significantly more distressed by this than the other two groups. Examining the burdens experienced, that is effects on the carer's physical and emotional health and on their social life and leisure time, reveals an overall significant difference between the groups but no individual group significant differences. However, the project carers were significantly less distressed by this than the day hospital carers. The greater level of support received by the project carers may be the main reason for these differences. A comparison of the malaise or stress score for the carers indicates that this was significantly lower for project carers than for those carers of elderly people in continuing hospital care. This confirms the observations of some studies which suggest that, although admission to care may reduce the practical burdens experienced by carers, it does not necessarily reduce feelings of anxiety and guilt associated with the admission (York and Calsyn, 1977; Smith and Bengtson, 1979; Challis and Davies, 1986; Stephens et al., 1991).

It appears, therefore, that the improvements in elderly people's well-being after discharge from hospital to the project were not achieved at the cost of higher levels of distress for their carers. Follow-up interviews six months later with project carers revealed no significant changes in any of these indicators, suggesting that the benefits experienced by the project carers appear to have continued over some time.

Table 4.4 indicates the costs of care over a six-month period. Two different figures are given for National Health Service costs because long-stay beds for elderly people in Darlington were mainly provided in an acute hospital, whereas elsewhere beds would be in a lower cost setting. The second, lower, cost estimate was based on the costs of the comparison group hospital. Even using the lower unit cost for hospital care, the most conservative assumption, there was an apparent cost advantage to the main agencies from the project. Social opportunity cost provides the most helpful comparison between the two groups, as it includes all the resources consumed in providing care, including costs to agencies, housing, personal consumption and private care costs. Even at the lower hospital cost, there still remains a significant cost advantage to the project of approximately £33 per week (p<0.001). This significant cost difference is not surprising given the comparison of the project

Table 4.4. Summary costs for different parties: price base 1986/87

	Over 6 months			Per week alive		
	Project £	Comprsn £	p value	Project £	Comprsn £	p value
The project	2850	–	–	143	–	–
Other SSD (revenue net cost)	29	115	–	1	4	–
Other NHS (5% capital allowance)						
DMH base[a]	870	9838	–	51	398	–
Geriatric base[b]	659	6204	–	39	251	–
Total agency cost						
DMH base[a]	3749	9953	<0.001	195	402	<0.001
Geriatric base[b]	3538	6320	<0.001	183	255	<0.001
Total public expenditure						
DMH base[a]	5084	9838	<0.001	259	398	<0.001
Geriatric base[b]	4873	6205	<0.001	247	251	ns
Total social opportunity cost						
DMH base[a]	5017	10493	<0.001	256	424	<0.001
Geriatric base[b]	4806	6859	<0.001	244	277	<0.001

'ns' = not significant.
a Long-stay hospital costs at Darlington Memorial Hospital (DMH) level.
b Long-stay hospital costs at geriatric hospital level.

service with the cost of long-stay hospital care, which would be expected to be more expensive than other forms of long-term care, either at home or in residential or nursing home care. However, these lower cost options would not have been a realistic alternative for the majority of elderly people who received the project service. (Further details of the analysis are presented in Chapter 9 of Challis et al., 1995.)

It is important, however, to move beyond looking at average costs to whether this service was cheaper or more expensive for clients with particular needs; that is, to look at targeting by trying to identify those individuals for whom the approach was likely to prove cost-effective. Cost predictions were made using the project service for various combinations of client and carer characteristics and circumstances, which proved to be significant determinants of variation in cost. As shown in

---

Box 4.1. Most and least costly types of case

Most costly cases

Risk of falling
Incontinence   } frequent assistance needed
Assistance needed with transfer
No carer or dependent spouse carer

Least costly cases

Less frequent assistance required
Carer not stressed
Carer undertaking several care tasks

Box 4.1, the most costly cases were those with particular health attributes which necessitated assistance on a frequent and regular basis: those who were at risk of falling, who were incontinent or who needed help with transfer. The most costly cases were also those with no carer, or those with a dependent spouse carer. Those cases who were least costly to the service were those who needed less frequent assistance, where the carer was not stressed or where the carer was undertaking several care tasks. It is clear that an efficient and effective service must provide adequate support for carers.

To conclude, it would appear that the greater benefits achieved for both elderly people and their carers in the project were at least no more expensive than the alternative provision of long-stay hospital care.

Implications of the Darlington study for policy and practice

A number of policy and practice implications for the development of community care and care management can be identified from the findings of the Darlington study (Challis et al., 1995). Of these, a number are specific to the need to achieve better linkages between health care and social care and the possible beneficial contribution of secondary health care services to community care. Four issues of particular concern may be identified:

- the integration of health and social care at the level of the hands-on worker;
- assessment, care management and secondary health care;
- the nature of care management in a specialised setting; and
- the location of care management.

Each of these is briefly considered below.

The integration of health and social care through the hands-on worker

One of the special features of the Darlington study was the development of the role of the home care assistant, which integrated the functions of home help, nurse aide and therapy aide into one person. The evaluation of the Darlington Project suggested that this was indeed a successful role model. Moreover, the development of such a role was recommended in the Griffiths Report, which was the precursor of the changes in community care arrangements in the UK (Griffiths, 1988). However, this role has developed in only a limited number of areas, and most of the developments would appear to have been predominantly health care-focused, with a specific orientation towards cost-effective alternatives to long-stay care. For example, a joint initiative between health and social care has been developed in the same social services authority where the original project was undertaken, and home care assistants are organised and employed by the social services (Peebles, 1989). The limited number of replications of this approach probably reflects at least two factors. The first is the relatively high cost of employing generic workers to undertake a range of tasks, some of which may be perceived to be activities which could be undertaken by less expensive employees. In the interests of the efficient use of staff, there is a clear temptation for agencies to avoid the possible overpayment of staff for some activities. Although, in terms of concerns of quality and effectiveness of care, it may be argued this is a false premise, in an era of constrained budgets it is readily possible to understand such a response by agencies. The second factor is closely related to this and is of course the boundary between health and social care. The very strength of the home care assistant function was that the individuals themselves undertook tasks which spanned the blurred boundary between the functions of nursing assistant, therapy aide and home help, a boundary which has itself been subject to marked shifts during the 1980s, as home care services have moved away from domestic care to concentrate upon personal care. From an agency perspective, the opportunity to benefit financially from a shift in the pattern of care provision can militate against even a jointly-purchased service, since not to collaborate may appear the least costly strategy. The later history of the Darlington service as it developed into a single-agency health care initiative demonstrates only too clearly these pressures, as described later in this book by Carr and Kelly, and elsewhere by Challis and colleagues (1995). It is clear, however, that at least for those clients requiring intensive amounts of care, the integrated approach offered by the home care assistant may be effective in avoiding potentially expensive care alternatives. The analyses from the Darlington study suggest that there are types of case for whom such an approach is particularly appropriate, as shown in Box 4.1. It would seem that if there is to be further development of the generic care worker then it must be focused upon clients with particularly intensive care needs. Such individuals might include the severely physically frail, those individuals suffering from dementia who need intensive care at home, the provision of terminal care or, as discussed later in this volume by MacMahon and colleagues, the provision of rehabilitation in the community. Despite the relatively few examples of generic workers, the evidence from the Darlington study is not that the role is inappropriate, nor that the organisational and budgetary inducements render it totally infeasible. However, such an approach must be clearly focused upon those individuals for whom an intensive approach to care delivered by relatively few care workers is most appropriate.

Assessment, care management and secondary health care

Since 1993 there has been considerable investment in the process of assessment, which has been cited as one of the cornerstones of effective community-based care (Cm 849, 1989). The Department of Health's own monitoring study of assessment procedures under the new community care arrangements suggested that assessments may often be variable in both form and content. Frequently, assessments were mono-disciplinary, rather than reflecting the multiple needs of individuals, with a consequence that insufficient NHS input has been provided to community care assessments, and particularly noteworthy was the lack of input from secondary health care services (Department of Health, 1993). It is worthwhile to consider the alternative approaches to assessment in community care from Australia, a country whose changes are particularly analogous to our own.

Australia was faced with a substantial growth in the provision of residential and nursing home care, led by a change in funding arrangements not dissimilar to that in the UK, which created a bias of provision towards institutional care. As in many countries, a major government initiative in the 1980s was undertaken to shift the balance of care. Under the new arrangements, residential and nursing home care was to be only a last resort for the most frail, reflecting their perceived preferences and also the sheer budgetary necessity of targeting scarce resources. As in the UK, resources were to be released for enhanced community services, in part using resources that had previously been invested in the provision of institutional care. Thus, at least three parallel elements in the organisation of Australia's Aged Care Reforms can be identified: improved assessment arrangements, enhanced provision of community-based services, and the development of coordination and case management. What was markedly different, and of particular interest in the light of the Darlington study, was the form of investment in assessment which was undertaken in Australia (Challis et al., 1995). The creation of Geriatric Assessment Teams ensured the provision of multidisciplinary assessment prior to placement in publicly-funded care settings. This has meant that initiatives related to the provision of long-term care, either in the community or in institutional settings, have involved secondary health care services and a very clearly prescribed role for geriatric medicine in the development of community-based care.

The effectiveness of these arrangements is of some interest. In the State of Victoria only 55 per cent of people referred for nursing home care were seen as needing a nursing home placement and subsequently placed there following multidisciplinary assessment. Those not placed received a variety of options such as enhanced community care and rehabilitation. Similarly, of those referred for residential care, again only 55 per cent were actually placed there, while others were diverted to alternative and more appropriate options (Otis, 1992). A similar study of the impact of geriatric assessment in Sydney, New South Wales indicated that only two-thirds of those referred for nursing home care were actually placed following geriatric assessment (Quartararo and O'Neill, 1990). The assessment process also appears to have contributed to improved targeting of those individuals entering nursing and residential care homes (Aged Care Research Group, 1993a,b), and Geriatric Assessment Teams appear to have assisted the development of broader roles for geriatric services in general (Ames and Flynn, 1992).

The outcomes of the Australian geriatric assessment approach, albeit one located in the broader context of a whole set of arrangements designed to shift the balance between community and institutional modes of care, parallels the evidence from studies of geriatric screening and assessment. These studies suggest that benefits include the detection of previously unrecognised disease and avoidance of inappropriate admission, as well as providing assistance in continuing management and support for very dependent elderly people (Brocklehurst et al., 1978; Rafferty et al., 1987; Kalra and Foster, 1989; Stuck et al., 1993; Peet et al., 1994). The development of a broader role for geriatric medicine and similar secondary health care services has not been formally explicated in the UK community care arrangements. In the light of the findings from the Darlington study, previous evidence about assessment and current concerns about assessment processes, it is worth considering whether the well-developed network of old age health care services in the UK could contribute more substantially to the provision of community-based care than at present with prevailing organisational incentives. The benefits may occur not only at the point of assessment, but also in the continuing management of vulnerable individuals in the community, and this is the other area where the Darlington Project raises interesting questions about the links between secondary health care and care management.

The nature of care management itself

The need for a differentiated response of care management for individuals with very disparate needs has been noted by Welch earlier in this volume. It seems self-evident that variations in the type and intensity of need require concomitant variations in the forms of care provided to meet those needs. This simple logic, paradoxically, seems at odds with some of the more generic forms of care management arrangements which have been developed (Department of Health, 1994). The model of care developed in the Darlington study was a form of intensive care management specifically designed for individuals with complex needs, for whom the level of risk was high and who, if coordinated and intense levels were not provided, would require costly forms of institutional care as an alternative.

If differentiated forms of care management are to emerge, then it might be organisationally appropriate for social services departments to discriminate between primary and secondary level responses. The SSI Guidance (SSI/SWSG, 1991a,b) discussed the provision of a care management approach for most individuals receiving services. There is no reason why this approach may not be differentiated in levels of intensity, with the majority of individuals being, as in health care, processed through a primary care system. Intensive care management (Challis, 1994) would then be a secondary process, to which only a limited and relatively small percentage of cases were referred, following initial screening and assessment. This would make social care arrangements parallel the forms of arrangements that occur in UK health care, with the majority of treatment and need provided for at a primary care level. Such a primary/secondary distinction may also help to identify with which settings it is most important for those undertaking the care management function to be linked, in order to undertake their work most effectively. Thus, it would be entirely logical for secondary-level responses, such as intensive care management for the physically frail elderly, to be linked with geriatric services, and for those supporting people suffering from dementia to be linked with old age psychiatry services. Such issues take us into questions of the most appropriate location for care management.

The location of care management

It follows from the proposition that intensive care management may be viewed as a secondary-level response, analogous to secondary health care, that the most appropriate location for care managers to work will vary depending on client group, form of care management and links with other professionals. For example, a primary-level response of care management, concerned with a wide range of needs and designed to improve case-finding as well as making effective links and complementary purchasing arrangements with GP fundholders, might most appropriately be located within a primary health care setting. However, there may be a much more appropriate case for linking intensive care management for physically frail older people with secondary health care settings such as geriatric medicine, particularly for assessment, complex care packages and monitoring of volatile needs. The evidence from Australia suggests that there are several advantages in linking care management with Geriatric Assessment Teams. A national evaluation of case management arrangements in Australia suggested that closer links between Geriatric Assessment Teams and case managers were particularly beneficial in dealing with incontinence, mobility problems and dementia (DHHCS, 1992). An additional benefit was that co-location also led to greater involvement of geriatric services in the mainstream community care system. The benefits in the Darlington Project of close links between care management and the geriatric service were in improved case-finding, and access to a wide range of skills in the assessment of need, not just initially but throughout the involvement with a client, including monitoring wellbeing. Thus, potential gains are evident, not only in the Darlington study but also in the Australian Aged Care Reforms, from linking care management with secondary health care provision (Gray et al., 1995).

Developing community care and secondary health care

Inevitably, the initial phase of instituting the community care reforms has been one of putting arrangements in place, and much of the concern of both health and social care agencies has focused upon sets of procedural directives. As arrangements settle down, and new changes occur — such as the reorganisation of local authorities, the further development of joint commissioning and consideration of more effective management of the health and social care interface — then a range of exciting opportunities may present themselves. At the macro level, arrangements such as single-agency provision may become more common, as has occurred in some areas in mental health care, with a trust employing health and social care staff. At the micro level, closer linkages between secondary health care and community care, including assessment, treatment, rehabilitation and continuing care at home, may similarly develop. The UK has made significant advances in the development of health care for older people and, as a consequence, has a substantial infrastructure and investment in this area. Now we are in an era of new opportunities where secondary care services may move away from a purely hospital-based focus, towards consideration of new forms of community-based health and social care for vulnerable older people. The considerations of the British Geriatrics Society (1994) in developing the role of community geriatricians may be just one precursor of this, and care management in secondary health care another. There is certainly room for exciting developments in intensive care management in secondary health care and the future is ripe for a range of valuable experimentation.

References

Aged Care Research Group (1993a) *Aged Care System Study: Eleventh Progress Report*, Lincoln Gerontology Centre, La Trobe University, Melbourne.

Aged Care Research Group (1993b) *Aged Care System Study: Twelfth Progress Report*, Lincoln Gerontology Centre, La Trobe University, Melbourne.

Ames, D. and Flynn, E. (1992) Dementia services: an Australian perspective, in A. Burns and R. Levy (eds) *Dementia*, Chapman and Hall, London.

British Geriatrics Society (1994) *Guidelines for the Role of Community Geriatrician*, British Geriatrics Society, London.

Brocklehurst, J.C., Carty, M.H., Leeming, J.T. and Robinson, J.M. (1978) Care of the elderly: medical screening of old people accepted for residential care, *The Lancet*, ii, 141-2.

Challis, D.J. (1994) *Implementing Caring for People: Care Management: Factors Influencing its Development in the Implementation of Community Care*, Department of Health, London.

Challis, D.J. and Davies, B.P. (1986) *Case Management in Community Care: An Evaluated Experiment in the Home Care of the Elderly*, Gower, Aldershot.

Challis, D.J., Chessum, R., Chesterman, J.F., Luckett, R. and Woods, R. (1988) Community care for the frail elderly: an urban experiment, *British Journal of Social Work*, 18 (Supplement), 13-42.

Challis, D.J., Chessum, R., Chesterman, J.F., Luckett, R. and Traske, K.J. (1990) *Case Management in Social and Health Care: The Gateshead Community Care Scheme*, Personal Social Services Research Unit, University of Kent, Canterbury.

Challis, D.J., Darton, R.A., Johnson, L., Stone, M. and Traske, K.J. (1991a) An evaluation of an alternative to long-stay hospital care for frail elderly patients: I. The model of care, *Age and Ageing*, 20, 4, 236-44.

Challis, D.J., Darton, R.A., Johnson, L., Stone, M. and Traske, K.J. (1991b) An evaluation of an alternative to long-stay hospital care for frail elderly patients: II. Costs and effectiveness, *Age and Ageing*, 20, 4, 245-54.

Challis, D.J., Chesterman, J.F., Darton, R.A. and Traske, K.J. (1993) Case management in the care of the aged: the provision of care in different settings, in J. Bornat, C. Pereira, D. Pilgrim and F. Williams (eds) *Community Care: A Reader*, Macmillan, Basingstoke and London.

Challis, D.J., Darton, R.A., Johnson, L., Stone, M. and Traske, K.J. (1995) *Care Management and Health Care of Older People: The Darlington Community Care Project*, Arena, Aldershot.

Cm 849 (1989) *Caring for People: Community Care in the Next Decade and Beyond*, HMSO, London.

Department of Health (1993) *Monitoring and Development: Assessment Special Study*, Department of Health, London.

Department of Health (1994) *Implementing Caring for People: Care Management*, Department of Health, London.

Department of Health, Housing and Community Services (DHHCS) (1992) *It's Your Choice: National Evaluation of Community Options Projects*, Aged and Community Care Division, Department of Health, Housing and Community Services, Australian Government Publishing Service, Canberra.

Department of Health and Social Security (DHSS) (1983) *Health Service Development: Care in the Community and Joint Finance*, HC(83)6, LAC(83)5, DHSS, London.

Davies, B.P. and Challis, D.J. (1986) *Matching Resources to Needs in Community Care: An Evaluated Demonstration of a Long-Term Care Model*, Gower, Aldershot.

Gray, L., Appleby, N., Farish, S. and Sullivan, M. (1995) *Bundoora Community Care Project, Evaluation Report*, Bundoora Extended Care Centre, Bundoora, Victoria, Australia.

Griffiths, R. (1988) *Community Care: Agenda for Action*, A Report to the Secretary of State for Social Services, HMSO, London.

Kalra, L. and Foster, C. (1989) Assessment of applicants for sheltered housing, *Age and Ageing*, 18, 271-4.

Otis, N. (1992) *Identifying Care Alternatives for Older People: The Victorian Regional Geriatric Assessment Program*, Lincoln Papers in Gerontology 13, Lincoln Gerontology Centre, La Trobe University, Melbourne.

Pattie, A.H. and Gilleard, C.J. (1979) *Manual of the Clifton Assessment Procedures for the Elderly (CAPE)*, Hodder and Stoughton, Sevenoaks.

Peebles, R. (1989) Diversion in Durham, *Community Care*, 27 July, Inside, vi.

Peet, S.M., Castleden, C.M., Potter, J.F. and Jagger, C. (1994) The outcome of a medical examination for applicants to Leicestershire homes for older people, *Age and Ageing*, 23, 1, 65-8.

Platt, S. (1985) Measuring the burden of psychiatric illness on the family: an evaluation of some rating scales, *Psychological Medicine*, 15, 2, 383-93.

Platt, S., Hirsch, S. and Weyman, A. (1983) *Social Behaviour Assessment Schedule (SBAS)*, 3rd edition, NFER-Nelson, Windsor.

Quartararo, M. and O'Neill, T.J. (1990) Nursing home admissions: the effect of a multidisciplinary assessment team on the frequency of admission approvals, *Community Health Studies*, 14, 441-9.

Rafferty, J., Smith, R.G. and Williamson, J. (1987) Medical assessment of elderly persons prior to a move to residential care: a review of seven years' experience in Edinburgh, *Age and Ageing*, 16, 1, 10-12.

Rutter, M., Tizard, J. and Whitmore, K. (eds) (1970) *Education, Health and Behaviour*, Longman, London.

Smith, K.F. and Bengtson, V.L. (1979) Positive consequences of institutionalization: solidarity between elderly parents and their middle-aged children, *The Gerontologist*, 19, 5, 438-47.

Social Services Inspectorate and Social Work Services Group (SSI/ SWSG) (1991a) *Care Management and Assessment: Managers' Guide,* HMSO, London.

Social Services Inspectorate and Social Work Services Group (SSI/ SWSG) (1991b) *Care Management and Assessment: Practitioners' Guide,* HMSO, London.

Stephens, M.A.P., Kinney, J.M. and Ogrocki, P.K. (1991) Stressors and well-being among caregivers to older adults with dementia: the in-home versus nursing home experience, *The Gerontologist,* 31, 2, 217-23.

Stuck, A.E., Siu, A.L., Wieland, G.D., Adams, J. and Rubenstein, L.Z. (1993) Comprehensive geriatric assessment: a meta-analysis of controlled trials, *The Lancet,* 342, 1032-6.

York, J.L. and Calsyn, R.J. (1977) Family involvement in nursing homes, *The Gerontologist,* 17, 6, 500-505.

5   The Darlington Service —
Past, Present and Future

Peter Carr and Sally Ann Kelly

As described in the previous chapter, the Darlington Community Care Project began in 1985 as a project funded for three years by central government under the Care in the Community Initiative. Since that time, it has continued as the Intensive Domiciliary Care Service (IDCS) with finances released from the closure of two long-stay wards in Darlington Memorial Hospital. During the following nine years or so of its existence it has cared for over 200 people, for whom the average length of service support has been about twenty months. Roughly one-third of the patients within the scheme have died at home and one-sixth in hospital, a tenth have been discharged from the scheme to a nursing home, and about the same number have improved sufficiently to be discharged to the care of the home help service. One-twentieth were readmitted into long-term care in hospital. At the time of writing, the scheme had places for 50 people.

The main objectives of the scheme were described in *Care Management and Health Care of Older People* (Challis et al., 1995). Briefly, these were:

- the maintenance at home of a group of physically disabled elderly people, who would otherwise have remained in long-term hospital care;
- the provision of both domestic and personal care by a single trained home care assistant, thus replacing the need for separate helpers;
- the quality of care and satisfaction of the client should compare

favourably with that of similar people receiving the more usual forms of care in hospital and the community;

- the cost of providing home care should compare favourably with that of long-stay hospital care; and
- to create an additional level of long-term care in the community for frail elderly people.

The evaluation of the project has suggested that all the objectives were met (Challis et al., 1995), but more recently a number of issues have been raised in connection with the operation, assessment and care management activities in the IDCS, and with aspects of its administration. Some of these issues have arisen out of the major changes that have occurred within the health and social services, both nationally and locally, and some are specific to the operation of the service itself. There are those that would argue that not all the changes have been for the good of the patient.

Implications of changes to health and social services

In 1985 the concept of an NHS trust was not even a speck on the horizon. Community and acute health care were run by a single authority. The number of nursing homes, although growing, was relatively small. The local authority provided the majority of home help, primarily for domestic reasons, and was also responsible for the majority of residential care. Community geriatrics was unheard of. There were many patients in hospital blocking beds while awaiting transfer to the continuing care wards.

However, the rapid increase in numbers of nursing homes provided a new source of care to which these patients could be transferred. Health authorities did not have to fund them. It became a relatively easy process to discharge patients, particularly those with little or no money, to nursing homes, with funding from the then Department of Health and Social Security. The assessments for these patients were of variable quality, depending on the source of referral. This diversity of assessments may have prevented some patients from being considered for the Darlington Project, for which the main factors limiting suitability appeared to be:

- the need for intensive night care;
- the degree of dementia; and
- the severity of disability, where the cost of more than one care assistant would preclude consideration for the scheme.

Substantial changes have now occurred. NHS trusts are now the norm, with many districts having separate acute and community units. Certain specialties in medicine, including geriatric medicine, have been faced with the choice of belonging to one or other of these units, and occasionally they may belong to both. Trusts are inevitably very cost-conscious, and currently continuing care in hospital is not a source of financial gain. As a result, there has been a very rapid reduction in the number of long-stay hospital beds throughout the country.

The former Department of Health and Social Security has split into two separate departments. The financial responsibility for the public funding of residents in residential and nursing home care, once the province of social security, now rests with local authorities. These authorities have a limited budget to provide for the community and institutional care of older people, and increasingly the care agencies are finding it very difficult to stretch these resources through the financial year. The hospital bed-blocker has returned and now there are some restrictions on the further closure of continuing care hospital beds (Department of Health, 1995).

There has been a changing role for social workers, some of whom have become care managers with greater powers of assessment, albeit sometimes done unilaterally. Local authorities and hospital trusts have an interest in preserving their own budgets, and the debate about health and social care sometimes leaves the patient in the middle as the loser. The role of the home help has changed too. He or she is now a 'home carer' concerned with personal rather than domestic requirements, the latter now being very much the province of the private sector.

Alongside these changes in the service environment were specific changes to the service itself.

The IDCS in operation

Organisational, management and service linkages

The operation of the Darlington Project is described in detail elsewhere (Challis et al., 1995). In 1988, at the end of the project, which was a joint health and social care initiative, the Intensive Domiciliary Care Service was established. The service was incorporated into the health service and was initially under the management of more than one manager, along with other services. There were three distinct organisational forms, affecting management, supervision and care management activities; furthermore, the incumbent of the post overseeing the care managers changed thirteen times in three years. From the end of 1991, the service continued to be managed within the elderly services unit by the elderly services manager, who was responsible for the day-to-day management of the service, in addition to responsibilities for the two acute wards, the two remaining long-stay wards (now closed), a day hospital and a community hospital. Therefore, senior management time available to the IDCS was greatly limited.

This left greater and wider roles for the two new service managers, who had been employed initially as administrative assistants, mainly dealing with the day-to-day activities of organising home care assistant rotas. They were expected to absorb the roles of care coordination and liaison with services, previously undertaken by others, for which they had not been trained. In their new roles, the new service managers began to deal directly with clients, carers and the allocation of tasks, and became directly involved with the referral, assessment and review procedures. Formalised support meetings with the teams of home care assistants became an important part of the support network, along with home visits to discuss care with clients and their families. The appointment of an administrative assistant relieved the service managers of much of the clerical work they had previously carried out themselves.

At present (1995), responsibility for the IDCS lies ultimately with the clinical services manager (a new management post created within the newly-formed South Durham Health Care Trust), who is also responsible for other services in the Darlington locality. The clinical services manager is also the budget-holder. This limits the level of response available to the service managers of the IDCS. Due to budgetary restraints, they do not have the flexibility to respond to needs as perhaps they feel they should or could. As it is provided by the NHS, the service continues to remain free of charge to its clients.

The staff of the IDCS have felt that this lack of stability in management has meant that, over time, those with budgetary control have begun to lose their appreciation of the service and its history of changes and, consequently, important areas have remained unclear in terms of responsibility. In fact, managerial oversight now appears to be detached from the service except in budgetary matters. Issues have arisen requiring decisive action, but it has been unclear who should take responsibility, each professional having responsibility solely for their own area. For example, on occasions, difficulties and conflicts have inevitably occurred between different elements in the care network, such as between carers and home care assistants. However, the current service managers have had insufficient authority to resolve these conflicts. On the one hand, they are not vested with sufficient authority by families and carers and, on the other, as non-professionals they are not respected by the different professional groups.

With the advent of separate NHS trusts, the IDCS has become increasingly separate from acute services, and thereby more isolated. Nonetheless, links with the acute unit, and indeed with the wider community, have been maintained to an extent through the service professionals, the consultant and, in turn, their links with their own peers. However, the disaggregation of the occupational therapy and physiotherapy services into smaller units has made this linkage difficult to maintain.

Closure of the remaining two long-stay wards has led to concern over the provision of respite beds. These constituted a major area of support to the service. Many clients have remained at home successfully with periods of respite care forming an important part of their support. The closure of the long-stay wards was an initial stage in the Durham Joint Commissioning Project, which is now considering the future management of the Intensive Domiciliary Care Service, along with other aspects of community care. Respite care continues to be provided for those clients already receiving it, but it remains to be seen whether the social services department is able to provide the degree of immediate crisis provision that was readily available on the long-stay wards. A related concern is whether the loss of respite care will, in time, increase pressure upon acute hospital beds as a means of relieving stressful situations and supporting carers at home. Certainly, both respite care and day care provision need to be considered hand-in-hand with daily home care assistant support. The maximum level of home care support is three visits per day, leaving long periods between calls, and it can only be a part of the means of providing adequate community support for many clients and their families. These clients have been assessed as requiring the level of care appropriate for nursing home placement, which offers 24-hour care, so it is a concern that further support is not available to cover the varying needs of elderly people within the community.

Within the last year, one of the two service managers retired, and it appears that no further appointment will be made to replace her. The service has also reduced the number of clients that it can comfortably support, within the constraints of the budget, to 50. Several home care assistants have either left, are unable to work due to long-term sickness or are on maternity leave. They have not all been replaced and so this has added pressure to the task of allocating sufficient care to clients, particularly the new referrals. Since a speedy response to referrals is essential, this may contribute to problems such as delaying hospital discharge or, indeed, slowing the introduction of the service to a prospective client in the community, thereby exacerbating any stress already being experienced.

Referral, assessment and review

Referrals from the hospital continue to be channelled through a consultant, while community referrals are channelled through GPs. Assessments to determine suitability are received from the physiotherapist, occupational therapist and district nurse, and forwarded for multidisciplinary team discussion with the service manager.

The criteria for client referral, in theory, have remained the same as when the project began: physically frail but mentally alert individuals over the age of 65 years. However, the interpretation of this has always depended significantly upon the client's individual needs and circumstances. More recently, the influence of health professionals and health needs has been the deciding factor for referral and acceptance of one case rather than another, as to a great extent similar, and equally dependent, individuals are receiving support from social services.

Communication links

Formal monthly review meetings are held to record any new referrals and discuss decisions regarding eligibility. The immediate members of the assessment team attend, as do the district nurses when they feel it is appropriate, depending upon the clients being discussed. Initially, multidisciplinary team meetings included a member from social services. However, a blurring of services over time meant that an element of territorial behaviour emerged. There was concern that social services would 'protect' their clients or 'poach' possible referrals. The service manager only becomes directly involved with the client and family once a client is accepted by the multidisciplinary team. Once agreement regarding family commitments is made, a contract is drawn up outlining each party's duties. This includes an agreement that the client may be transferred to another, more appropriate service if a change in circumstances arises. This move from health to social services care inevitably imposes a charge on the client.

A care plan and daily time sheet are kept in the client's house, allowing all care assistants and visiting professionals to pass on information relating to the client's care. Basic issues such as bowel routine, catheter care and handling difficulties can be noted. This system helps to ensure a greater degree of continuity and consistency of care. Care assistants also contact each other directly to pass on information that appears to be inappropriate to leave written on the time sheet. The care plan outlines information regarding a client's daily routine and care procedure, so that any care assistant is clear about the tasks to be undertaken.

Following acceptance, clients receive a six-weekly review to ensure that their needs are being met. Following this, reviews are conducted on a nine-monthly rota rather than six-monthly, as formerly, since for many clients their situation appeared to remain fairly static for several months at a time. Any changes or problems relating to a client are brought forward to the next review meeting to allow more immediate discussions. Home care assistants attend the reviews of their particular clients, to relay information regarding their present care, changes in circumstances and how they feel the client and their family are coping. However, in most cases the assessment team is made aware immediately of any changes in a client's situation, and the review meeting merely formalises issues. The service manager is not directly involved in the review, other than to receive the information from the multidisciplinary team and implement any decisions taken. This may involve visiting the client and family to discuss changes in the care plan.

There are also informal weekly discussions between service managers, community health staff and home care assistants and, of course, telephone contact is maintained daily, together with home visits where appropriate. Bi-monthly meetings of the four teams of home care assistants are organised and supported by the service manager.

Risk assessment

An area of importance within the IDCS has been the continuous training and support given to the care assistants. Areas covered include auxiliary nursing skills, pressure care, catheter care, and handling and lifting techniques.

The introduction of EC guidelines regarding handling and lifting placed a duty of assessment of risk upon employers, and led to the development of a risk assessment package by the therapists involved in the service. In the case of new referrals this has meant merely a formalisation of procedures which were already carried out. With current clients the assessment examined existing practices, usually assessing those situations which seemed to cause most problems. These usually arose as a result of changes in a client's condition or related circumstances. The assessment aimed at identifying risk in the areas of environment, handling of the client and equipment used. Over the years the service has been running, the identification of need for equipment, and also the carers' attitudes towards using it, have changed dramatically. In the very early days the home care assistants were often reluctant to use a hoist. They disliked the extra time it took, preferring to lift manually, often putting themselves and possibly the client at risk. However, by carefully assessing risk and providing appropriate equipment and training, the quality of care provided and the accompanying level of safety may be improved. In addition, the standard of equipment available has improved considerably over the last ten years, but the cost, and sometimes a delay in purchasing it, has proved at times to be very frustrating. Clients' needs change over time and are therefore reassessed. This has implications for the provision of appropriate equipment: for example, specialist beds, mattresses and handling equipment.

The importance of appropriate and detailed assessment can be illustrated by the case of a woman being cared for by social services. Her needs changed considerably and substantially more physical help was required. The initial, single-discipline assessment led to the provision of inappropriate equipment and inadequate training and support for home care staff. The client was subsequently referred to the IDCS by her GP, and she was assessed and accepted by the service through the multi-disciplinary process. Although there were difficulties in caring for this client, they were overcome and her husband commented that the approach of the IDCS was 'more professional'. This example illustrates that a difficult situation can be managed well, given access to a range of assessment resources and follow-up support, and shows the type of case for which the service was particularly suited.

The IDCS and social services

By virtue of the changes in the service and its environment, much of the assistance provided by the IDCS and the local authority now have many similarities, so it could be asked whether real differences remain. Perhaps the best way to illustrate the differences is to look at the roles of the care staff themselves and the operation of the scheme. For the purposes of the discussion, care staff from the domiciliary care scheme will be referred to as care assistants and those from the local authorities as home care staff.

- The care assistants receive a series of lectures and training on a variety of subjects related to their role, including talks on basic personal care, lifting and transferring, skin care, cardiopulmonary resuscitation, and dressings. Regrettably, in very recent years these lectures have become rather more sporadic. Perhaps this is because of the rapid turnover in the higher levels of management of the scheme so that no one has been in post long enough to tackle the situation or to understand its workings. Nonetheless, such health-related training is rare for social services home care staff.

- There is also some training on a one-to-one basis with the individual client and care assistant. This comes from a variety of sources, including paramedical staff and district nurses. The care assistant may well be asked to do some basic nursing care such as dressings or supervising the administration of drugs. Again, this one-to-one training is rare for social services home care staff.

- The time care assistants are able to spend with their clients is rather more flexible than that of home care staff. Home care staff have a very rigid timetable, sometimes spending as little as fifteen minutes with one person before going to see another. Care assistants will take as long as seems to be necessary, although the average time per week spent with each of their clients is just over fifteen hours. They become key workers with individual clients, unlike social services home care staff.

- The mode of admission to the domiciliary care scheme is through a full multidisciplinary assessment. This involves medical input as well as that from physiotherapy and occupational therapy staff and a district nurse. At one time a social worker was also involved, but unfortunately this is not now the case. In contrast, community-based schemes appear to be developing without adequate medical and paramedical input (Department of Health, 1994a). The gains from a multidisciplinary assessment team do not seem to have been learned. Access to home care provided by social services is rarely through such a multidisciplinary process.

- The care plan for a client within the IDCS is drawn up and agreed between the service, the client and his or her relatives. It is reviewed regularly at a multidisciplinary meeting, depending upon changes in the client's circumstances. Reviews have often posed problems for home care (SSI, 1987; Department of Health, 1994b).

- The IDCS remains a free service to the client, the funding coming from the community trust. At one time, respite care was also free in the remaining continuing care wards, although the families of new clients requiring respite will have to pay for provision from social services, with potential effects on their willingness to use the service. The social services home care provision is subject to charging.

Thus, certain distinctions remain between the IDCS and social services domiciliary support with regard to the care of elderly people, particularly the link with health care professionals, but it may be that some form of merger will occur. The change in emphasis in the role of the home help towards providing personal care around the time the project ended created an overlap between the two services. This overlap has become greater and more blurred over time, and no doubt it will have an effect on the development of the Intensive Domiciliary Care Service, and it may be that the service itself will influence and reinforce changes in social services.

The closure of the long-stay wards, the implementation of the 1990 NHS and Community Care Act and the formation of a community trust do not seem to have created an appropriate setting for the IDCS within the health service. Furthermore, the service seems to be rather isolated, as it also lacks the formal links with the social services network necessary to be able to respond appropriately to a client's wide range of needs. Again, a tightening of the budget available for the service has reduced flexibility.

A recent example regarding the care of a client of the IDCS illustrates some of the limitations of the service and its isolation. A marked change occurred in a client's needs, as so often happens. A second care assistant was required because a hoist was thought to be inappropriate for lifting. Night care was also required, and the client's carer had needs which required support. All of these requirements could not be met within the IDCS budget and, indeed, for cost reasons clients could only be cared for on a one-to-one basis. In order to purchase extra care for both client and carer, a care manager from social services was involved. This, however, created an unsatisfactory working situation, with different care workers from different agencies attempting to work together, all with different training standards, providing fragmented care. This led to confusion regarding the overall management and responsibility for the total package of care.

An element in the success of the domiciliary care scheme has been the ongoing support and training to home care assistants provided by health professionals. This has also allowed a continuation of rehabilitation, or at least maintenance therapy, within the service. Particularly in the light of recent EC regulations regarding manual handling and lifting, it is imperative that appropriate assessment, training, equipment and support mechanisms are available to ensure a quality service is provided for all those involved. However, rehabilitation has, as yet, hardly featured on the social services agenda.

The social services department has made links with the health services through GP practices, by allocating care managers to primary health care. By responding to those patients requiring more intensive support, it is likely that health and social services can support each other in providing community care. For example, the assessment and support provided by health professionals to care assistants in the community and links with the geriatric service were elements in the Darlington Project that helped it to be so successful, and can be seen as examples of a positive way forward in joint working practices.

The future of the IDCS

The IDCS started out as a joint collaborative scheme. Over the years local authority involvement has declined, and the service is currently provided by the community trust. Once it was relatively easy to obtain extra help and services when required, whether from social services or other parts of the NHS. This is not now the case, and a major concern is whether the IDCS will become isolated and less effective.

The infrastructure of the service appears to lend itself to development in a number of directions. One would obviously be rehabilitation, and there have been a number of patients in the scheme who have been discharged to less intensive forms of service. An obvious comment might be that these particular patients were insufficiently dependent for the service in the first place, but the average time spent in the scheme for these patients was ten months, which may indicate otherwise. Paramedical services are available for any client within the scheme, although not on a regular basis, and currently there is no qualified occupational therapist. Nevertheless, there is obviously scope for rehabilitation at home, either as part of the continuing management of the patient from an acute unit, or perhaps for patients for whom rehabilitation at home would offer an alternative to hospital admission. A second possible development would be 'hospital at home'. This could provide a service similar to that operating in Peterborough (Mowat and Morgan, 1982), and could be used either to prevent admissions or to facilitate earlier discharge from hospital. It could also be suitable for an unexpected crisis at home.

Another group of clients poorly provided for are the young chronic sick. Very few facilities exist in the locality for this group. There are two clients in this category among the 50 currently supported by the IDCS. These clients were admitted at the time when the service was not fully subscribed, and it was never the intention to develop this aspect of the service further since it would have clearly reduced the number of places available for elderly patients. The terminally ill have also occasionally been included in the scheme. The locality now has a developing hospice movement, and there is no reason why the two services could not benefit each other. There might also be a case for including those people who require night care. The biggest problem in providing this greater intensity of care has always been the cost.

It is worth considering organising a scheme within the acute unit, similar to that of the Intensive Domiciliary Care Service, with a view to identifying those patients who could benefit from early discharge from hospital but who still required a degree of rehabilitation and auxiliary nursing support. Such a form of short-term support would not necessarily require the involvement of the social services department, which is much more necessary when considering the longer-term needs of elderly people.

For the IDCS to move forward as a service able to care for severely physically dependent elderly people within the community, it needs to be able to provide a specialist service with a range of care provision equivalent to that provided within a nursing home. At present, there is no provision available for those clients requiring two care assistants, no formal provision for crisis situations when an additional care assistant is required, and no provision for additional visits appropriate to a client's needs. Intensity of support has been reduced. However, it does have the framework for offering a good support and training system, although stronger management is needed to give the required support to the service managers and the service as a whole. Using its existing organisational arrangements within a wider social services network, and with the continuing involvement of health care professionals, the Intensive Domiciliary Care Service could continue to offer a quality service to those dependent elderly individuals who wish to remain living in their own homes.

Two questions remain to be answered: 'Who runs the scheme?' and 'Who pays for it?' A community geriatric service, with experience in multidisciplinary assessment and organisation, could be a very attractive candidate to run the service, particularly if it were extended in any of the directions indicated above. Such a service would need strong links with and influence upon the acute hospital unit, local authority and other services so as to be able to provide more seamless care.

In its present form, in 1995, the average cost of the service per client, worked out purely in terms of the total budget for the service and the number of clients covered, amounts to about £230 per week per client. This is little different from the cost of a similarly-run private service elsewhere in the locality. Should it continue to be a free service to the client, and what would the implications be for all potentially interested parties? The philosophy of the National Health Service was, at its inception, to provide free care from the cradle to the grave. The economic argument against a free IDCS is obvious. The political argument would perhaps revolve around what constitutes 'health care'. It is not the remit of this chapter to discuss these points. However, if the arrangements concerning nursing home admission were applied, and the IDCS was regarded as 'nursing home at home', the client would be expected to contribute something to his or her care. This amount might be topped up as necessary by either the health authority or the local authority. This could, of course, lead to difficult discussions between the two budget-holders, and such a situation begs the development of a single budget-holder within a district for health and local authority long-term care services. Perhaps the funding for the service could be regarded as a loan to the patient, and the home itself used as collateral at a later stage.

The rising number of elderly people, more and more of whom may be appropriate for the IDCS or other community-based schemes, is evident from demographic data or, indeed, can be seen from within a service. Not all will be able to afford their own care, and local authorities are experiencing difficulty now in coping with the numbers. Will there be enough money in the future? One partial solution might be to encourage the public to invest in its own future from a much earlier age, say eighteen, with tax-exemption schemes which will provide the funds for care when and if it becomes necessary. Long-term care insurance raises many complex questions.

If the IDCS were to develop in different directions, there would be implications for other services. For example, a 'hospital at home' service may mean that fewer beds would be needed in an acute unit. However, any beds closed would be spread over a number of wards, rather than one, thus limiting the amount of money saved. In practice, therefore, any new form of service is likely to cost more money overall.

In summary, the Darlington Intensive Domiciliary Care Service has been successful in providing a new quality care service for elderly patients in the spirit of the NHS and Community Care Act. The multi-disciplinary initial and continuing assessments have been vital to the wellbeing of the client and fundamental to its success. Its basic structure lends itself to development in a number of directions and perhaps might best be controlled by a community geriatric service with footholds in all care provider units from the acute hospitals to the local authorities and through a strong, stable management structure. A single budget for health and social services would have distinct advantages when organising or developing a community service such as this. However, it is unlikely that any government will have enough funds to meet the needs of dependent elderly patients and there will have to be some attractive schemes in the future to enable members of the general public to save for their future care in old age.

References

Challis, D.J., Darton, R.A., Johnson, L., Stone, M., and Traske, K.J. (1995) *Care Management and Health Care of Older People: The Darlington Community Care Project*, Arena, Aldershot.

Department of Health (1994a) *Implementing Caring for People: Community Care Packages for Older People*, Department of Health, London.

Department of Health (1994b) *Implementing Caring for People: Care Management*, Department of Health, London.

Department of Health (1995) *NHS Responsibilities for Meeting Continuing Health Care Needs*, HSG(95)8, LAC(95)5, Department of Health, London.

Mowat, I.G. and Morgan, R.T.T (1982) Peterborough Hospital at Home Scheme, *British Medical Journal*, 284, 641-3.

National Health Service and Community Care Act 1990 (1990 c. 19) HMSO, London.

Social Services Inspectorate (SSI) (1987) *From Home Help to Home Care: An Analysis of Policy, Resourcing and Service Management*, Social Services Inspectorate, London.

6 Assessment and Rehabilitation Teams in the Community: The Cornwall Experience

Douglas MacMahon, Christine McKee and Ken Buckingham

The radical reforms that have occurred in the health and social services during the early 1990s have many implications for the management of elderly and disabled people in the community. First, the community care arrangements enacted in April 1993 assume a multidisciplinary assessment of needs. The health input into this process was not clearly defined, and therefore has been implemented variably around the country. However, it is widely recognised that such an assessment, and the therapeutic actions that are suggested by that assessment, are clearly necessary, particularly for those whose independence is threatened. This is especially so for those persons who are on the threshold of admission to institutional (residential or nursing home) care. Second, the increasing pressure upon hospital inpatient beds has led to increasing difficulty in admitting patients for non-acute conditions, and earlier discharge of rehabilitating patients, with a consequent shift of need, but not usually resources, to the community. Unnecessary permanent admission to nursing or residential care is sometimes the unfortunate result of pragmatic placement. The concept of Community Assessment and Rehabilitation Teams (CARTs) has arisen as a result of these themes, in order to complement existing specialist services, particularly in geriatric medicine and medical rehabilitation. A pilot project evaluating the implementation and efficacy of two such teams was established in the County of Cornwall. This chapter describes the findings of the pilot scheme and the conclusions drawn about the efficacy of this approach that have led to its further local development. From our experience of the first year of its operation, we suggest further developments that may be required for wider implementation.

Rationale

Disabled persons are at their most vulnerable when struck by a social crisis, a new medical insult, or by the progression of chronic disabling disease. In addition to the physical morbidity, they are also delivered to the threshold of admission to institutional care, that is, admission to hospital, a residential or a nursing home. It was implicit in the NHS and Community Care Act 1990, and the white papers that preceded it, that recipients of care, particularly those at public expense, should have a full assessment of their needs by a fully-trained specialist team at the most vulnerable time of their lives. The statutory requirement is described in the White Paper *Caring for People*, which recommended that:

> All agencies and professions involved with the individual and his or her problems should be brought into the assessment procedure when necessary. These may include social workers, GPs, community nurses, hospital staff such as consultants in geriatric medicine, psychiatry, rehabilitation and other hospital specialties, nurses, physiotherapists, occupational therapists, speech therapists, continence advisers, community psychiatric nurses, staff involved with vision and hearing impairment, housing officers, the Employment Department's Resettlement Officers and its Employment Rehabilitation Service, home helps, home care assistants and voluntary workers. (Cm 849, 1989, para. 3.2.5.)

The method for obtaining this multidisciplinary assessment was to be locally determined, through the care management process. Clearly, it is a major challenge for all health service providers from primary and secondary care to provide this assessment, and a major problem for social services, as the lead agency, to organise such a process. We question how this has been addressed through the length and breadth of the country, since anecdotal evidence is that it is at best patchy and at worst non-existent.

The present structure of health and social services, with separate lines of funding, different accountability and variable models of interagency and interprofessional working, is undoubtedly an obstacle to seamless care. Although it is implicit in the NHS and Community Care Act that social services shall be the lead agent in arranging community care, it is now apparent that in order to meet their financial targets for supporting care in the community, many fewer places will be funded in nursing and residential homes. The corollary will be that more people will remain in their own homes, requiring pan-agency support from health, social and private provider units.

Although these arrangements should lead to a more flexible approach to caring for people with disability, particularly in old age, there is an urgent need to establish systems to ensure effective assessment procedures leading to appropriate care packages to support people in their own homes, or appropriate and timely admission to hospital, for rehabilitation if required, before assuming that permanent admission to nursing or residential care is necessary.

In addition to the statutory requirements upon the health and social agencies for assessment, there is the important question of the rights of the individual to receive appropriate care. Those rights are spelt out by the World Health Organization, which defines the need for rehabilitation:

> By the year 2000, people with disabilities should be able to lead socially, economically and mentally fulfilling lives with the support of special arrangements that improve their relative physical, social and economic opportunities (World Health Organization, 1991).

The other major factor influencing the need for community rehabilitation arises from the increasingly rapid utilisation of acute hospital facilities and the reduction in the overall number of hospital beds, with the associated reduction in the length of each inpatient stay. The 'Efficiency Index' may also drive health commissioners and the health providers (mainly trusts) to seek ever-increasing throughput, hence earlier discharges. The other possibility (which has been widely feared but has yet to be demonstrated) would be a tendency to avoid admission of patients with more complex conditions, with the potential requirement for more lengthy inpatient treatment because of their need for rehabilitation. The increased pressure upon community resources suggests that a review of the placement of valuable rehabilitation staff is now required (Squires, 1994).

There are two distinct responsibilities in our present system. While health agencies have the lead responsibility for treatment, social services departments have the statutory responsibility to assess need and to ensure the supply of care (i.e. support). The distinction between 'therapeutic' and 'prosthetic' models of intervention essentially corresponds to this difference in responsibilities. True multidisciplinary assessment will encompass both of these threads in a well-woven tapestry.

Health service responsibilities

The prime responsibility for accessing health care lies with general practitioners and the primary health care teams. The general practitioner is clearly in a central coordinating position, and their involvement is the key to the provision of effective community care.

Trusts are charged with the provision of secondary care, and have responsibilities to ensure that they have adequate liaison with GPs and the primary health care team which they undertake in a variety of ways. Some have well-developed liaison services, and others have developed outreach services. In the market economy that health services have now entered, purchasers (both health and social services) need to be persuaded of the positive contribution of such input, as measured by outcome criteria such as 'QALYs' and 'health gain'. However, such methods may discriminate against elderly people, and also against their carers who may, indirectly, be greater beneficiaries of health and social care than the elderly people themselves.

Both purchasers (or commissioners) and providers have a legitimate clinical and managerial interest in seeing the best utilisation of resources. Purchasers will require adequate safeguards to ensure that limited resources are best targeted, while providers will need to clarify their responsibilities to avoid either duplication or service shortfalls. Both will need to ensure that contracts are set appropriately, and obtain the necessary activity information to satisfy the monitoring of those contracts.

Social services responsibilities

Care management is a relatively new discipline for many departments. A perception has developed that the specialist role has been devalued to a more generic one. However, the best examples of practice, such as that of McEvoy and colleagues in York (A. McEvoy, personal communication), have attached social workers to hospital and community-based specialist teams, and similar models of good practice have been noted elsewhere, such as in reports by the Health Advisory Service.

The responsibilities of the social services have been clarified since their central role in community care was identified in Sir Roy Griffiths' report (Griffiths, 1988), and subsequently have been enshrined in law with the NHS and Community Care Act 1990. They now have the responsibility, but do they have the necessary skills?

The process of placement in a residential or nursing environment inevitably entails major changes of lifestyle and, to a variable degree, the loss of privacy, the loss of independence and, most feared, the loss of dignity. While it is undeniable that many elderly or disabled people welcome admission to care, many dread it. For those who do wish to enter care, and cannot have their needs met otherwise, entry should be facilitated provided the resources are available. However, every effort should be expended at the point of referral to retain independent living for those who do not wish to enter care, but want instead to remain in their own homes in their natural community.

There is an extensive body of literature demonstrating the benefits of a full multidisciplinary assessment at the point of entry to care, and there is also evidence showing the inappropriate nature of some admissions to institutions. For example, Brocklehurst et al. (1978) identified significant new medical conditions among 80 per cent of the entrants to residential care in their study. They demonstrated evidence of misplacement, and suggested that 27 per cent could be found more appropriate alternatives to residential care and 16 per cent could stay at home with support. This indicates that, for a substantial minority, the chance to avoid institutionalisation would have been missed without skilled input. The medical assessment led to frequent referral to therapy departments, chiropody and other modalities of care. In a similar study, Bradshaw and Gibbs (1988) found that 17 per cent of residential care dwellers could have been cared for in their own homes.

The absence of specialist input into the care of individuals admitted to nursing homes may also result in mismanagement of the, often complex, needs of this client group. Hepple et al. (1989) showed injudicious use and control of medication among the nursing homes of Weston-super-Mare. We have data that not only corroborate this, but also suggest that there was evidence of misplacement in a nursing home in which residents were supported by the Department of Social Security prior to the changes in 1993 (MacMahon and Maguire, 1993). Better placement decisions were evident in a group of patients selected and managed by a multidisciplinary team, in terms of disability, mental and physical handicap, nursing care of pressure areas, and drug use.

The role of the hospital in support of community care has perhaps received little emphasis, other than a concentration on discharge arrangements. In particular, the professional input into services for older people, including their mental health, merits further consideration. We would contend that facilities must change and develop to accommodate the reducing length of hospital stay. Taking a typical admission of a hemiplegic patient, the medical needs are at their greatest at the onset of the stroke, but dwindle with time. Similarly, nursing needs change, with a reduction in supportive compensatory care and a move towards a re-enablement mode of care. This is where physiotherapists and occupational therapists often have their maximum input. Speech therapy may need to continue for many months. Squires (1994) has portrayed this variation in staff activity patterns through time graphically, as shown in Figure 6.1. Suitably trained and skilled professionals are in short supply, and we are continually reminded of financial restraints. If expansion is not feasible, the corollary of shorter hospital stays for these patients must be a shift from hospital-based and closeted therapy staff, with relatively narrow roles, towards greater input in the wider community. In so doing, care must be taken to avoid any reduction of professional standards among the community multidisciplinary team.

Lastly, hospitalisation is often the final factor precipitating permanent entry to care. Although a minimal length of stay in hospital is clearly desirable, it should not be at the expense of re-admission. Post-discharge intensive support has been demonstrated to improve the chances of effective return to the community, and avoid the penalty induced by a failed discharge, which severely compromises the chance of a further successful discharge.

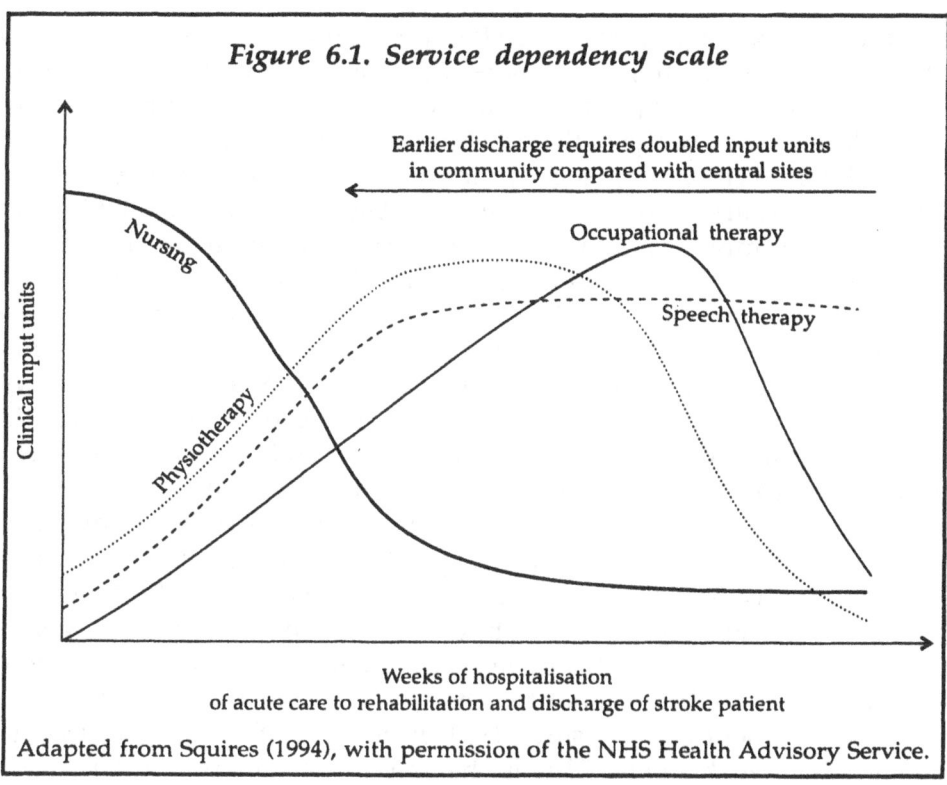

Figure 6.1. Service dependency scale

Earlier discharge requires doubled input units in community compared with central sites

Occupational therapy

Nursing

Speech therapy

Physiotherapy

Clinical input units

Weeks of hospitalisation of acute care to rehabilitation and discharge of stroke patient

Adapted from Squires (1994), with permission of the NHS Health Advisory Service.

Solutions

A new method of working has been advocated by many authorities, including the Audit Commission. Essentially, the needs of the patient or client should be central to, and dictate, the way in which resources are deployed, and the resources should be accessible from a single point of contact. In many ways this is the ethos behind many departments of geriatric medicine, which should strengthen their traditionally strong links with social services since their efforts are largely synergistic. Anecdotally, relationships have become less close since the introduction of the 1990 Act, but we hope that this reflects more upon the managerial challenges associated with change and the financial culture, rather than exposing a major structural fault line developing between these key agencies.

Before embarking upon the CARTs pilot project, we first ascertained the views of general practitioners and community staff, and found evidence of strong support for the concepts of community care, but also a lack of knowledge of the processes that would support it. Looking around for examples of good practice in assessment, we found the model of Geriatric Assessment Teams in Australia (Gregory, 1992), and also a community hospital-based procedure in the United States (Applegate et al., 1983). The experience of the Australian teams has been particularly impressive, having shown that significant savings can be made in the nursing home placement budget from a marked reduction in a previously uncontrolled flood of admissions to nursing homes. We understand that the programme has now moved on to look at ways in which community rehabilitation can be developed (Central Sydney Area Health Service, 1994; G. Broe, personal communication).

Closer to Cornwall, Community Rehabilitation Teams in Tavistock and Plymouth have been shown to provide effective rehabilitation in the community, and we acknowledge their assistance in the establishment of our own project. Dr Gabrielle Greveson, a community geriatrician in Newcastle, is also developing a community team approach, based upon a medical model that has evolved towards a multidisciplinary assessment process since 1974. It entails both aspects of assessment and re-enablement. This is the essence of the approach that we have taken in forming CARTs, which we will explore in more detail in the rest of this chapter.

Method

The remainder of this chapter describes the evaluation of a pilot project of Community Assessment and Rehabilitation Teams in Cornwall. This was a joint project between the Cornwall Healthcare Trust, Cornwall and Isles of Scilly District Health and Family Health Service Authorities, Cornwall County Council Social Services Department, and Tor and South West College of Health Studies. It was funded through joint funding in the year 1993-94 and the evaluation was completed during 1994-95.

The first and main aim of the CARTs project was to examine how the community assessment and rehabilitation needs of disabled and elderly people could best be met. It was anticipated that this should be through better deployment of existing resources, ensuring a fit with the care management process in the production of care packages, and augmented with selective development of targeted rehabilitation resources in the community.

A second aim of this study was to supply both purchaser and provider management organisations with periodic information to feed into their business plans to allow for more effective provision of health care, to complement that provided by the social care agencies, private sector providers, and primary care teams in support of community care.

The referral criteria were as follows:

- Patients who have a major need for rehabilitation in order to help them remain in their own homes.
- Patients who have a particular problem with daily living activities which need to be addressed at home.
- Patients for whom early discharge can be facilitated by community rehabilitation.
- Patients who require multidisciplinary assessment prior to entry to a nursing home.
- Patients who require interventions to prevent hospital admission, including nursing assessment of complex needs, respite care and carer support.

Access to the team was designed to be simple and effective, i.e. by telephone or fax referral, and a generic approach was adopted to avoid territorial disputes. Communication between team members, GPs and social services has been central to the successful introduction of the project.

Following a period in which existing facilities and manpower were reviewed, the two pilot locations were selected for their demographic profile, the lack of existing community resources, and subject to the agreement of local management. Staff were appointed initially to short-term contracts, and a period of training and orientation was organised. In each site, the staffing amounted to one whole-time equivalent (WTE) physiotherapist and a 0.5 WTE occupational therapist, supported by a 0.5 WTE clerical assistant. These staff worked alongside the existing eldercare specialist nurse (geriatric liaison nurse) and consultant geriatrician in each of the two areas.

As part of the evaluation, a controlled trial was attempted. The characteristics of the trial and control subgroups are shown in Table 6.2, below. The control subjects were drawn from referrals to social services in areas other than those which were served by CARTs teams. They were selected in the expectation that they would be of similar dependency to the trial group. Permission was sought to include all suitable referrals to these control areas. Consent was obtained from the local research ethics committee, and informed written consent was obtained from all subjects included in the trial.

Efficacy was judged by several methods. Admissions to all forms of institutional care were identified, including residential and nursing homes and hospital; and the Barthel score (Royal College of Physicians and British Geriatrics Society, 1992) was used as an index of dependency. A survey of referral agencies was performed, and a patient and carer satisfaction survey was undertaken. Tolerance was assessed by the effect upon morale and stress levels in the patients, and their caregiver strain (Robinson, 1983). Changes within the two groups were examined over six months.

Results

The project was formally evaluated. In the first year, 473 cases were referred to the teams. The rate of referral was brisk. The baseline data are shown in Table 6.1. Although the majority of referrals were elderly, a small but significant number were much younger, but needing the same team approach. Many of the younger referrals were carers of other disabled relatives, and their support at time of need was indicated in order to prevent not only their own admission, but also that of the relative for whom they were caring.

Table 6.1. Demography of referrals

	Range	Mean
Patient age (years)	18-99	77
Carer age (years)	20-92	65
Barthel score	0-20	14.0

Number of referrals = 473.

Table 6.2. Characteristics of trial and control recruits

Variable	CARTs	Control
Male (%)	27	35
Age (mean)	78.3	70.1*
Barthel score (mean)	14.6	15.8
Morale score (mean)	9.9	10.0
Norton score (mean)	16.1	16.3
Living alone (%)	24	9
Incontinent (%)	17	7
Caregiver Strain (mean)	6.0	5.3
Number of cases	59	26

* $p < 0.05$

The progress of the controlled trial was adversely affected by very slow recruitment to the control group, partly because of withheld consent, and partly through non-compliance with the interview schedule. There were no statistically significant differences between the two groups (see Table 6.2) other than in age, where the trial (CARTs) patients were significantly older. There was a trend for the trial patients to be more dependent and more incontinent, their carers exhibited greater levels of strain, and more lived alone than the controls; however, none of these differences reached statistical significance.

There was a trend for the CARTs patients to remain at home, in comparison to the controls (p=0.08), as shown in Table 6.3. The Barthel score was used as an index of dependency, and showed no significant overall change in either group, as shown in Table 6.4. A smaller subgroup for whom rehabilitation was the goal showed evidence of the efficacy of the rehabilitation process. A survey of referral agencies confirmed anecdotal accounts of individual success stories. A reduction in carer strain was seen only for the CARTs patients, and not for the controls (Table 6.4).

Finally, a patient and carer satisfaction survey was performed. A significant improvement in satisfaction with services was observed for patients in both control and intervention groups, but among carers the improvement in satisfaction was only significant in the CARTs group. Patient and carer satisfaction scales undertaken by a source independent of the CARTs team (social services) corroborated the trial findings.

Table 6.3. Location before and after intervention

Variable	CARTs				Control			
	Before		After		Before		After	
	No.	%	No.	%	No.	%	No.	%
Home[b]	40	82	41	84	17	89	15	79
Institution[c]	8	16	8	16	2	11	4	21
Other	1	2	–	–	–	–	–	–
Total	49	100	49	100	19	100	19	100

a Overall significance of locational changes: $p = 0.08$.
b Includes with relative or friend, and warden-controlled accommodation.
c Includes nursing home, residential home and hospital.

Table 6.4. Physical and psychological outcomes

Variable	CARTs			Control		
	Before	After	No.	Before	After	No.
Barthel score	15.12	15.78	50	15.68	16.00	19
Morale score	10.06	9.86	47	11.42	10.86	17
Caregiver Strain	6.25	4.80*	20	3.25	2.75	4
Patient satisfaction	2.37	4.24*	45	1.82	4.38*	17
Caregiver satisfaction	3.41	4.59*	17	4.25	4.75	4

* $p < 0.05$ (After:Before)

Carer strain decreased for 60 per cent of patients treated, increased for 35 per cent, and remained the same for 5 per cent.

We may therefore conclude from this pattern of results that the CARTs intervention was popular with patients, and especially with carers, among whom there was evidence of a reduction in stress.

Discussion

This was essentially a pilot study. The statistics are not robust, the numbers are small and there were a variety of confounding issues.

Notably, implementation took place at a time of major change in both health and social services, with the care management changes wreaking huge management change in the latter, and the formation of a new trust from the merger of a trust with two directly managed units (DMUs) in the health service.

Nonetheless, we are confident that the data support the hypothesis that trained, targeted staff deployed in the community can assess, and then support, appropriate people in their own homes. It is encouraging to note the reduction in carer stress. The lack of change in the Barthel score is not surprising since the referrals were from a severely disabled group, many of whom would not be expected to improve, and also because of the lack of sensitivity of the scale to relatively small changes. A larger population in both intervention and control groups would be required to establish statistical proof of these findings, and we would encourage researchers to continue this line of enquiry.

Organisational issues that have arisen from this work, and also in other projects, include the management of the greater workload for the physiotherapy and occupational therapy professions, the nature of the inter-professional relationships of the team, and the tightness of the definition of the referral criteria. Most projects find they are unable to handle a long-term caseload, since they are very committed with new referrals. Some limit the length of intervention to a certain number of visits, others to a maximum time period. As in the analogous 'hospital at home' schemes, the possibility of using multitasking generic helpers, both in the short term and for longer-term support, is being considered.

Many of the patients, carers and professionals were confused about the roles of support agencies, and found difficulty in distinguishing the CARTs team members from other health or social agency staff. Evidence of team work was difficult to demonstrate: for example, only 8 per cent of visits were joint. However, it was felt that the teams were working in a delegated fashion, and were responding to need in an appropriate way. The teams would usually pick the most appropriate member to handle a referral, who would discuss it with other team members on returning to base. The lack of understanding of the role of CARTs team members in relation to other community professionals has led us to the view that the 'CARTs' function should be one function of an integrated team, rather than that of a separate team. In the full implementation we plan to base the teams locally, and the majority will be based in a community hospital, fulfilling another function of these units (Royal College of General Practitioners, 1990).

The role of the nurse in the team has led to some conjecture. The specific nursing interventions of the liaison nurse were few, and their role in the CARTs team appeared to be somewhat nebulous. We are attracted to other models in which nurses have taken on a care management role, particularly for those clients who would appear to be similar to those referred to the CARTs project.

Our study is by no means the only example of such work linking assessment and rehabilitation. Indeed, we have already alluded to work in Devon, Newcastle and York. However, when searching for published material in this area, we found a paucity of well-validated research. Other schemes have also found that training needs were underestimated, particularly for those staff with little or no previous community experience. Despite this handicap, the teams worked well with general practitioners, hospital consultants, care managers and other community staff. Interviews with each of these groups showed high levels of satisfaction with the CARTs service.

Conclusions

The advent of the NHS and Community Care Act 1990 has demonstrated the need for multidisciplinary assessment of needs. The specialist health input into this process needs to be examined. It is particularly necessary for those persons who are on the threshold of institutional care, those for whom discharge from hospital is likely to be difficult, and direct referrals from general practitioners of patients with ill health who wish to remain in their own homes. It needs to be multidisciplinary, coordinated and locally appropriate, drawing on existing strengths, which should be augmented where necessary.

We have appointed two pilot teams consisting of an occupational therapist and a physiotherapist along with clerical support, which complement local primary and secondary care services. Linking the assessment with skilled rehabilitation appears to be a logical development which is effective, well tolerated and popular with both patients and their carers. There was evidence of reduction in carer stress, and reduced institutional admission of patients. In addition to the trial findings, anecdotal evidence supports both the concept of CARTs and its method of working.

The CARTs model, as described in this chapter, provides access for disabled people to a specialist team and appears to provide an appropriate solution for the local circumstances in Cornwall. Further work is required to demonstrate the efficacy of this approach elsewhere.

Acknowledgements

The Cornwall Healthcare Trust.

Cornwall and Isles of Scilly District Health Authority and Family Health Service Authority.

Cornwall County Council Social Services Department.

Tor and South West College of Health Studies.

Especial thanks to the CARTs team members, and local health and social services staff for their cooperation.

The project was funded by Cornwall and Isles of Scilly District Health and Family Health Service Authorities by a grant from Joint Finance.

References

Applegate, W.B., Akins, D., Vander-Zwaag, R., Thonik, A. and Baker, M.G. (1983) A geriatric rehabilitation and assessment unit in a community hospital, *Journal of the American Geriatrics Society*, 31, 206-10.

Bradshaw, J. and Gibbs, I. (1988) *Public Support for Private Residential Care*, Avebury, Aldershot.

Brocklehurst, J.C., Carty, M.H., Leeming, J.T. and Robinson, J.M. (1978) Care of the elderly: medical screening of old people accepted for residential care, *The Lancet*, ii, 141-2.

Central Sydney Area Health Service (1994) *Strategic Directions*, Central Sydney Area Health Service, Sydney, NSW.

Cm 849 (1989) *Caring for People: Community Care in the Next Decade and Beyond*, HMSO, London.

Gregory, R. (1992) *Aged Care Reform Strategy: Mid Term Review 1990-1991*, Australian Government Publishing Service, Canberra.

Griffiths, R. (1988) *Community Care: Agenda for Action*, A Report to the Secretary of State for Social Services, HMSO, London.

Hepple, J., Bowler, I. and Bowman, C.E. (1989) A survey of private nursing home residents in Weston Super Mare, *Age and Ageing*, 18, 1, 61-3.

MacMahon, D.G. and Maguire, R. (1993) *Evaluation of Nursing Home Patients in Contracted DHA Beds*, Unpublished Research Report, Barncoose Hospital, Redruth, Cornwall.

National Health Service and Community Care Act 1990 (1990 c. 19) HMSO, London.

Robinson, B.C. (1983) Validation of a Caregiver Strain Index, *Journal of Gerontology*, 38, 3, 344-8.

Royal College of General Practitioners (1990) *Community Hospitals – Preparing for the Future*, Occasional Paper 43, Royal College of General Practitioners, London.

Royal College of Physicians and British Geriatrics Society (1992) *Standardised Assessment Scales for Elderly People*, Royal College of Physicians of London and British Geriatrics Society, London.

Squires, A. (1994) Key issues for purchasers and providers in hospital, day hospital and community rehabilitation services for older people, in NHS Health Advisory Service, *Comprehensive Health Services for Elderly People*, NHS Health Advisory Service, Sutton, Surrey.

World Health Organization (1991) *Targets for Health for All*, World Health Organization, Geneva.

7 Standardised Assessment in the Community

Iain Carpenter

As societies develop, their populations age, and, as health services become more sophisticated, expectations rise and so do costs. As expectations rise and hospital activity changes, there is growing interest in who is admitted and who is discharged. The earliest population health indices used readily-available numerical indicators such as mortality rates. As societies evolve, health problems alter in salience, and new health indicators must be chosen to reflect changing health issues: the resolution of one health problem casts new issues into prominence and reduces the usefulness of the prevailing health indicator, necessitating its replacement by others (McDowell and Newell, 1987). Indicators of hospital service activity have also evolved from simple Hospital Activity Analysis (HAA) information to the more sophisticated requirements of today, which include recently published Department of Health Performance Tables, Health Care Resource Use Groups (HRGs) (Information Management Group, 1994), and Health Status and Health Benefit Groups (HBGs) being developed by the National Casemix Office (NCMO). The same processes are now underway in community care. More people with complex needs live in the community and they require complex health and social service support programmes to maintain them in their own homes. The key to the understanding of their needs and the evaluation of their care requirements lies in information from comprehensive assessment.

Assessment in the UK context

Concern about assessment in the UK has come to the fore following the implementation of the NHS and Community Care Act 1990, with the greater focus upon outcomes in the purchase of care. Earlier work on assessment took the form of refining the content of assessment and monitoring tools (see, for example, Challis and Chesterman, 1985), and was also concerned with issues of appropriacy of placement (Brockle-hurst et al., 1978; Hutchinson et al., 1984). The focus of such work was upon the content of assessment and improving its quality by norms of professional practice. However, there has been a growing concern to consider the use of more reliable and valid indicators, and the possibility of using some standardised scales for outcome measurement and to provide comparable information across facilities, organisations and settings (Royal College of Physicians and British Geriatrics Society, 1992). Most recently in social care, the advent of the community care reforms has led to a massive investment in procedures and modes of assessment to implement the reforms more effectively. Much of this was based on high levels of laudable local effort, but was without reference to work undertaken elsewhere and, as a result, the re-invention of the wheel was inevitable.

As part of a programme to monitor the implementation of community care, the Social Services Inspectorate undertook a study on assessment procedures during 1993 (Department of Health, 1993), intended to identify examples of good practice and to examine issues for development. The study found that there was a great deal of variation in the content and quality of the documentation examined. The quality of categorisation of needs and problems was poor, with a tendency to focus on describing rather than analysing need, and there was a lack of reliability and validity in the information collected. Also, it was felt that there were too few health care staff involved in assessment which, as a consequence, was often monodisciplinary. Generic documents, where one complete assessment form was used for all adults, were seen as too vague, while the documentation in general was considered too long and complex. There was also a lack of clarity about the purpose of the assessment record: whether it was mainly for agency accountability, a guide for the assessor, to inform the user, for service planning, or some combination of these. Finally, there appeared to be no clear linkage between the identification of problems and the formulation of responses. Most notable, however, was that these assessments focused predominantly on the initial concern of the social services with the implementation of community care, namely the placement of older people and the construction of intensive packages of care for needy individuals. Several of these observations were confirmed in more local studies, which raised the importance of the relationship between assessment documents and the requisite skills and training (Caldock, 1993), and also noted the concentration of focus in assessment tools upon the functional domains and financial aspects, with consequently less focus upon others (Caldock, 1994).

Effective assessment in the community

Comprehensive assessment must take account of the extent to which needs cross disciplinary boundaries, and any documentation must be usable in routine practice. Numerous assessment scales with specific purposes, such as activities of daily living (ADL) scales and depression rating scales, have been devised for use in research with elderly people and people with disabilities. Some have passed into routine clinical use. However, the variety of scales and the variability of their use in practice makes comparisons between patients very difficult. As mentioned earlier, the British Geriatrics Society and the Royal College of Physicians recently recommended a number of scales for routine use, in a document entitled *Standardised Assessment Scales for Elderly People* (1992). However, completing a number of scales, or using an instrument compiled from a number of others, may lead to problems when assessing a person. For example, items may overlap. Where there are two almost identical items, choosing the preferred one should not be too difficult, but where two items are similar but test slightly different areas, separating the questions or choosing one rather than the other will not be as straightforward. Furthermore, instruments devised predominantly for research may not transfer easily into routine day-to-day practice. A well-structured, validated and integrated data collection system, designed to cover all the domains required for comprehensive geriatric assessment, could have distinct advantages over systems developed from compilations of others.

A wide range of professionals work in the community to maintain people in their homes. Each has their own area of expertise and, although they communicate between each other, they provide their services separately. Different people have different requirements, and so the input from the variety of professionals will vary according to those requirements. Huxley, in the following chapter of this book, discusses the different functions of the spotter, assessor and specialist roles, and describes how a professional who is a spotter for one client, may be an assessor or specialist for another. In order to provide an optimum level of care, a professional working with a client must be able to identify problems which lie in the domain of another professional.

An example of how the current arrangements may lead to assessors omitting factors that need to be addressed is given in a study by Buckley (1989), who examined the information gathered by different professionals assessing the same clients. In his study, short video clips and a brief history of elderly people were presented to different professionals. One such video clip showed an elderly lady who had fallen and was climbing some stairs, clearly in pain. The social work assessor was very interested to know of her support networks and who would be there to help her if she could no longer manage the stairs. The district nurse was very concerned about the pain, thinking about how it should be managed, and the health visitor was concerned about why she had fallen, and was interested in the medication she had been taking. The emphases of these assessments were very different and the likely consequent interventions similarly different, and were probably only partial in relation to the elderly person's needs.

Uses of assessment information

Ideally, information collected during assessments should be useful to a variety of people. It is helpful to consider assessment information as having value at different levels, from individual care planning to strategic planning. A tick sheet which satisfies the needs of the assessor alone has limited application. The assessment must involve both the client and the carer, so that they are informed about what is being done, and what is likely to be the outcome. Clearly, an assessment tool needs to be useful to the immediate assessor, guiding them towards good practice, but it also needs to generate information useful for managers. Anyone managing a service needs to know the range of needs of their population.

Planners and policy-makers at more strategic levels also need to be informed, using more aggregated information. Currently, social services departments, who have the responsibility for assessment in the community, are all developing their own assessment protocols, all of which may have good features but which are all different from each other. At regional and national levels, decisions cannot currently be based on comparable information because of the disparate nature of the information from the different assessments. At this final level the information should also be useful for research. Research based on standardised information permits comparisons of different interventions and different patterns of service provision, and thereby enhances the growth of knowledge.

The depth and focus of assessment

Not only does the information need to have relevance for different purposes, but it needs to be useful to both the health and social services, since complex needs require health and social service interventions. Ideally, the information should be shared between the two services in order to avoid duplication. These requirements put considerable demands on the assessment process. A further requirement is to contribute to the identification of the effectiveness of interventions.

Currently, it remains difficult to distinguish why it is that one group of people does better than another under different forms of provision. This requires the measurement of outcomes. There are examples of outcomes of care in the Darlington Project (Challis et al., 1995), and in the work of CARTs teams described by MacMahon et al. in the previous chapter of this book. The measurement of outcome is dependent upon high-quality baseline measures. However, although it is possible to gather information on what people are like at the beginning of a care programme and on what they are like at the end, we have little idea of what is going on in the middle (that is, during the work of the rehabilitation or care team). The care plan provides the necessary linkage between assessment and outcome. Following assessment, problems are identified, the means of whose resolution needs to be explicitly formulated into a care plan. This provides a clear strategy to move towards desired outcomes by specifying the necessary stages of intervention.

Ideally, then, an assessment done by one professional should be of use to another. The assessment should cover the domains relevant for intervention by each of the agencies working in the community, and ideally should lead to the same identified needs, whichever professional undertakes it and wherever it takes place. There should be no reason why a person living in one district should not have the benefits provided by another. Or, if there is a difference, it should not be on the basis of a different assessment of need, but on a difference in policy regarding available resources. It is only through undertaking assessments of a similar form that one can begin to understand the differences in client populations and determine the service requirements of those populations. The recent government guidelines on long-term care (Department of Health, 1995) address this point. Of course, there must be the possibility of appeal against decisions made on the basis of an assessment, and hence the grounds for those decisions must be accessible.

It follows, therefore, that assessment instruments should be standardised and reliable, allowing for reproducible assessment on different occasions and in different areas, usable by health and social services, able to provide comparisons of outcome as well as need, and should be related to a recorded care plan which is accessible for audit purposes. These ideal requirements for a community-based assessment are shown in Box 7.1.

Available assessment instruments

A recent survey of assessment documents in use in the UK confirmed the work of the Social Services Inspectorate and others, described earlier in this chapter. It indicated that the variability of assessment documents was high and that their comparability and their capacity to generate standardised information were low (Challis et al., 1996). Although a number of standardised assessment instruments are available — such as the Clifton Assessment Procedures for the Elderly (CAPE) (Pattie and Gilleard, 1979) and the Crichton Royal Behaviour Rating Scale (CRBRS) (Wilkin and Jolley, 1979) — these have limited application

---

Box 7.1. Requirements for ideal community assessment of elderly people

Assessment needs to be standardised	To ensure all domains are covered
	To maintain consistency
	To ensure a proper record
	To ensure a proper record for future reference
	To ensure a proper record to support decisions made
	To enable comparisons to be made
Information needs to be useful	The client and carer(s)
	The user
	The manager
	The planners and policy-makers
	The researcher
Assessment usable by health and social services	Information shared
	Meet health and social service needs
	Avoid duplication
Enable comparisons of process and outcome	Linkage between the assessment and the intervention
	The care plan

---

since they do not include a number of important domains such as an assessment of mood and social support. Wide-scale implementation of standard approaches is rare and probably requires policy leadership. One example of this process is the Minimum Data Set/Resident Assessment Instrument (MDS/RAI), developed in the United States for use in institutional care (Morris et al., 1990).

The Minimum Data Set/Resident Assessment Instrument (MDS/RAI)

In the United States, following scandals and reports of poor-quality care in institutions, the Health Care Financing Administration (HCFA) proposed a revision of regulations and procedures for ensuring quality of care. As part of this, the need for resident assessments in long-term care settings led the HCFA to develop a uniform resident assessment system. The goal of this exercise was to produce an instrument with a core of items necessary for comprehensive assessment of nursing facility residents linked to assessment protocols, and a structured framework for organising assessment elements that could be used to inform the care planning process (Morris et al., 1990).

The MDS/RAI has two components: the Minimum Data Set (MDS) and the Resident Assessment Protocols (RAPs). The MDS is a collection of data items covering all the domains commonly used in assessing the elderly and developing a care plan. It is completed as an admission assessment and then periodically during the course of institutional care. The RAPs are a series of protocols which guide the assessor through the best practice of care planning for the common problems faced by elderly people. They specify trigger items within the MDS which are conditions that may warrant a care planning intervention: for example, that a person has a current problem. Triggers consist not only of single items, such as incontinence of urine, but also of more complex com-binations. Thus, people who are extremely physically dependent have one set of care needs, and people who are severely cognitively impaired have another, but those who are both cognitively and severely physically impaired can have a totally different set of care plan requirements. The triggers identify not only existing problems, but also areas where there is risk of developing a new problem in the absence of preventative intervention, for example risk of pressure sores. They are also designed to identify where a person has particular strengths that would benefit from rehabilitative interventions.

The MDS/RAI is a multidisciplinary assessment which was designed to address problems of quality of care in nursing homes in the USA, but it is also being evaluated in a number of countries around the world. It is used on admission to homes and then on subsequent reviews of residents. Its use has improved the accuracy of completion of assessment forms and improved the accuracy of assessment and care planning, and has reduced admissions to hospitals from nursing homes and has had an impact on the outcome of care (Phillips, 1994). As explained above, where the assess-ment identifies a problem it triggers an assessment protocol which guides the assessor through good practice to develop a care plan for the identified problem. In this way it gives the user a return for its use while gathering reliable standardised data for the evaluation of care. The same principles are now being applied to the development of a home care assessment tool.

The RAI-Home Care (RAI-HC)

The RAI-HC was designed on the same principles as the MDS/RAI, as shown in Box 7.2. It is a home health care extension of the MDS/RAI, and has the same structure. It is being developed by an international group of researchers and clinicians in elderly care, pooling experience from several countries with a wide range of health and social service structures, to develop a standardised assessment and enable cross-national comparisons (Morris et al., 1997). Like the MDS/RAI, the assessment has a system of triggers. If a problem is identified during the course of assessment, a Client Assessment Protocol (or CAP) is triggered

---

Box 7.2. The RAI-HC

Structure	Standardised assessment
	Developed by interRAI, an international group of clinicians and researchers, MDS-HC is the assessment instrument
	Assessment items trigger Client Assessment Protocols (CAPs)
	CAPs guide assessor through best practice in developing a care plan
Development	Panels of 'experts' in each domain
	Review of relevant literature
	CAPs based on specified framework
	Triggers for each CAP are assessment items
	Field testing of reliability and validity
Uses	Usable by health and social service professionals
	Allows for analysis of problems, care plans and interventions
	An educational instrument
	Inter-district and cross-national comparisons

to guide the assessor to the best practice in developing a care plan.

Development of the RAI-HC

Development of the RAI-HC began with identification of the domains important for managing people at home. Panels of individuals with expertise in those areas then set about designing the CAPs for each domain. The work began with a literature review of each subject area to obtain the latest research and practice information. The CAPs were then constructed according to a standard framework, consisting of specified objectives, clear triggers, background and care planning guidelines. The objective of the CAP is to define the nature of the problem and the course of action to be undertaken. The 'triggers' frame the questions required to identify the problem to be included in the assessment, and to trigger the CAP. The background describes the nature and epidemiology of the problem and, finally, the guidelines provide descriptions and supplementary questions to be used to develop an appropriate care plan for that problem. The guidelines can be thought of as a checklist to ensure that all factors that could be causing the problem, or which might be suitable for an intervention to relieve the problem, are included or considered in the care planning process. Once the CAPs were written, they were sent for review to individuals for comment on the adequacy of the content and structure.

The assessment instrument was then constructed around the trigger items defined within the CAPs. The instrument is now complete and being tested for reliability and validity to complete the scientific development process.

Content of the RAI-HC

There are 30 different assessment protocols which cover a whole range of possible problems, including social, mental, physical and medical problems. These are listed in Box 7.3. There are CAPs to identify people who would benefit from rehabilitation, such as those helped by the CARTs initiative (see MacMahon et al., in this volume); people with anxiety and depression, which are often unrecognised; and people with

---

Box 7.3. Client Assessment Protocols of the RAI-HC

Adherence	Instrumental ADLs
ADL/rehabilitation potential	Medication management
Alcohol abuse and hazardous	Nutrition
drinking	Oral health
Behaviour	Pain
Bowel management	Palliative care
Brittle support system	Preventive health measures:
Cardio-respiratory	immunisation and screening
Cognition	Pressure ulcers
Communication disorders	Psychotropic drugs
Dehydration	Reduction of formal services
Depression and anxiety	Skin and foot conditions
Elder abuse	Social function
Environmental assessment	Urinary incontinence and
Falls	indwelling catheter
Health promotion	Visual function
Institutional risk	

---

brittle support systems. A brittle support system exists when a new or relatively small problem would precipitate the breakdown of the support system and lead to admission to an institution. Another CAP addresses the question of reducing formal services when a person's condition has improved or goals have been met, reflecting the need for review identified by the Social Services Inspectorate (1995).

Appendix 1 reproduces the assessment instrument, the RAI-HC. It is more structured than many assessment instruments. Information recording is based on a 'tick box' design rather than a large area for free text, to enable systematic comparisons. Each item has a specific definition of the area addressed and then a small area for recording. This allows for easy entry into a computer to form a database and all the benefits that accrue from that (Carpenter and Bernabei, 1995). Areas for free text can be incorporated into the instrument, but much of the free text is restricted to the care planning part of the procedure where such highly individual material is crucial.

Appendix 2 reproduces the Falls CAP. It offers an illustration of the structure of a CAP. The one shown covers background factors relating to falls, defines the problem, and gives a description of areas that are important to and may contribute to falls. The CAP lists risk factors systematically, covering both intrinsic and extrinsic aspects of the problem, and provides a comprehensive discussion of factors that need to be addressed when developing the relevant aspects of a care plan for someone who has been prone to falling. The CAP does not provide the care plan, but takes the assessor through best practice in developing the care plan. The structure of the assessment and the assessment protocols means that it can be used as an educational instrument. Being trained in its use leads to a better understanding of the health and social problems faced by many elderly people, and the way in which these should be managed.

Conclusion

Assessment, when standardised and linked to care planning, as described above, can make a measurable difference. It needs to be structured and standardised to be reliable, and to provide comparable results. The results need to be usable by both health and social service professionals. The health service professionals doing the assessment have to remember and consider the things that the social worker would spot, and vice versa. The assessment has to be structured in a way that allows for the analysis of problems, the analysis of outcomes and what happens in between. The RAI-HC has many of these characteristics and has exciting potential, covering the domains of health and social care and enabling inter-district comparisons. With the growth of such instruments, the possibility of comparing people with the same problems, and comparing the quality, outcome and cost of their care, becomes a reality. In a climate where concern is developing over the plethora of assessment tools available, further testing of this standard tool is relevant to the needs of policy and practice in community health and social care.

References

Brocklehurst, J.C., Carty, M.H., Leeming, J.T. and Robinson, J.M. (1978) Care of the elderly: medical screening of old people accepted for residential care, *The Lancet*, ii, 141-2.

Buckley, E. (1989) Health assessment of the elderly at home, Unpublished MD Thesis, University of Edinburgh, Edinburgh.

Caldock, K. (1993) A preliminary study of changes in assessment: examining the relationship between recent policy and practitioners' knowledge, opinions and practice, *Health and Social Care in the Community*, 1, 3, 139-46.

Caldock, K. (1994) The new assessment: moving towards holism or new roads to fragmentation?, in D. Challis, B. Davies and K. Traske (eds) *Community Care: New Agendas and Challenges from the UK and Overseas*, Arena, Aldershot.

Carpenter, G.I. and Bernabei, R. (1995) Database needs and practical models: is a minimum data set or common database possible and/or desirable?, in L.Z. Rubenstein, D. Wieland and R. Bernabei (eds) *Geriatric Assessment Technology: The State of the Art*, Editrice Kurtis, Milan.

Challis, D.J. and Chesterman, J.F. (1985) A system for monitoring social work activity with the frail elderly, *British Journal of Social Work*, 15, 2, 115-32.

Challis, D.J., Darton, R.A., Johnson, L., Stone, M. and Traske, K.J. (1995) *Care Management and Health Care of Older People: The Darlington Community Care Project*, Arena, Aldershot.

Challis, D.J., Carpenter, I. and Traske, K.J. (1996) *Assessment in Continuing Care Homes: Towards a National Standard Instrument*, Personal Social Services Research Unit, University of Kent, Canterbury.

Department of Health (1993) *Monitoring and Development: Assessment Special Study*, Department of Health, London.

Department of Health (1995) *NHS Responsibilities for Meeting Continuing Health Care Needs*, HSG(95)8, LAC(95)5, Department of Health, London.

Hutchinson, P., Evans, J. Grimley and Greveson, G. (1984) Linking health and social services: the liaison physician, in J. Grimley Evans and F.I. Caird (eds) *Advanced Geriatric Medicine 4*, Pitman, London.

Information Management Group (1994) *What are Version 2 Healthcare Resource Groups?*, NHS Management Executive, London.

McDowell, I. and Newell, C. (1987) *Measuring Health: A Guide to Rating Scales and Questionnaires*, Oxford University Press, Oxford.

Morris, J.N., Hawes, C., Fries, B.E., Phillips, C.D., Mor, V., Katz, S., Murphy, K., Drugovich, M.L. and Friedlob, A.S. (1990) Designing the national resident assessment instrument for nursing homes, *The Gerontologist*, 30, 3, 293-307.

Morris, J.N., Fries, B.E., Bernabei, R., Steel, K., Ikegami, N., Carpenter, I. and Gilgen, R. (1997) *RAI-Home Care (RAI-HC) Assessment Manual. Primer on Use of the Minimum Data Set-Home Care (MDS-HC) Version 10a and the Client Assessment Protocols (CAPs)*, interRAI Corporation, Washington, DC.

National Health Service and Community Care Act 1990 (1990 c. 19) HMSO, London.

Pattie, A.H. and Gilleard, C.J. (1979) *Manual of the Clifton Assessment Procedures for the Elderly (CAPE)*, Hodder and Stoughton, Sevenoaks.

Phillips, C., Hawes, C., Mor, V., Hines, M., Morris, J., Fries, B. et al. (1994) *Implementing the Nursing Home Resident Assessment Instrument: The Nursing Home Industry's Response to Mandated Assessments*, Research Triangle Institute, North Carolina.

Royal College of Physicians and British Geriatrics Society (1992) *Standardised Assessment Scales for Elderly People*, Royal College of Physicians of London and British Geriatrics Society, London.

Social Services Inspectorate (SSI) (1995) *The Social Services Contribution to the Rehabilitation of Older People*, Report of Conference, July 1995, Department of Health, London.

Wilkin, D. and Jolley, D. (1979) *Behavioural Problems among Old People in Geriatric Wards, Psychogeriatric Wards and Residential Homes 1976-1978*, Research Report No. 1, Research Section, Psychogeriatric Unit, University Hospital of South Manchester.

Appendix 1

The MDS-HC assessment instrument, Version 10a

MINIMUM DATA SET - HOME CARE (MDS-HC)©

(Status in last 7 days unless other time frame indicated—Note, if less than 7 days since last assessment, code all items that reference last 7 days on the basis of status since last assessment)

SECTION AA. NAME AND IDENTIFICATION NUMBERS

1.	NAME OF CLIENT	a. (Last/Family Name)	b. (First Name)	c. (Middle Initial)
2.	CASE RECORD NO.			
3.	GOVERN-MENT PENSION AND HEALTH INSURANCE NUMBERS	a. Pension (Social Security) Number		
		b. Health insurance number (or other comparable insurance number)		

SECTION BB. PERSONAL ITEMS *(Complete at Intake Only)*

1.	GENDER	1. Male 2. Female
2.	BIRTHDATE	Month Day Year
3.	RACE/ ETHNICITY	1. American Indian/Alaskan Native 4. Hispanic 2. Asian/Pacific Islander 5. White, not of 3. Black, not of Hispanic origin Hispanic origin
4.	MARITAL STATUS	1. Never married 3. Widowed 5. Divorced 2. Married 4. Separated 6. Other
5.	LANGUAGE	Primary Language 0. English 1. Spanish 2. French 3. Other
6.	EDUCATION *(Highest Level Completed)*	1. No schooling 5. Technical or trade school 2. 8th grade/less 6. Some college 3. 9-11 grades 7. Bachelor's degree 4. High school 8. Graduate degree
7.	RESPONSI-BILITY/ ADVANCED DIRECTIVES	a. Client has a legal guardian 0. No 1. Yes
		b. Client has advanced medical directives in place (for example, a do not hospitalize order) 0. No 1. Yes

SECTION CC. REFERRAL ITEMS *(Complete at Intake Only)*

1.	DATE CASE OPENED/ REOPENED	Month Day Year
2.	REASON FOR REFERRAL	1. Post hospital care 4. Eligibility for home care 2. Community chronic care 5. Day care 3. Home placement screen 6. Other
3.	WHERE LIVED AT TIME OF REFERRAL	1. Private home/apt. with no home care services 2. Private home/apt. with home care services 3. Board and care/assisted living/group home 4. Nursing home 5. Other
4.	WHO LIVED WITH AT REFERRAL	1. Lived alone 2. Lived with spouse only 3. Lived with spouse and other(s) 4. Lived with child (not spouse) 5. Lived with other(s) (not spouse or children) 6. Lived in group setting with non-relative(s)
5.	PRIOR NH PLACEMENT	Lived in a nursing home at anytime during 5 years prior to case opening 0. No 1. Yes
6.	RESIDEN-TIAL HISTORY	Moved to current residence within last two years 0. No 1. Yes

SECTION A. ASSESSMENT INFORMATION

1.	ASSESS-MENT REFERENCE DATE	Date of assessment Month Day Year
2.	REASONS FOR ASSESS-MENT	TYPE OF ASSESSMENT 1. Initial assessment 2. Follow-up assessment 3. Routine assessment at fixed intervals 4. Review within 30-day period prior to discharge from the program 5. Review at return from hospital 6. Change in status 7. Other

SECTION B. COGNITIVE PATTERNS

1.	MEMORY	Short-term memory OK — seems/appears to recall after 5 minutes 0. Memory OK 1. Memory problem

☐ = When box blank, must enter number or letter   ⬚ⓐ = When letter in box, check if condition applies

MDS-HC Draft 10a — 05/09/97
©Copyright interRAI Corporation, Washington D.C., 1994,1996, 1997   MDS-HC - Pg 1

2.	COGNITIVE SKILLS FOR DAILY DECISION-MAKING	How well client made decisions about organizing the day (e.g., when to get up or have meals, which clothes to wear or activities to do) 0. INDEPENDENT—decisions consistently reasonable 1. MODIFIED INDEPENDENCE—some difficulty in new situations 2. MODERATELY IMPAIRED—decisions poor; cues/supervision required 3. SEVERELY IMPAIRED—never/rarely made decisions
3.	INDICATORS OF DELIRIUM	a. Sudden or new onset/change in mental function (including ability to pay attention, awareness of surroundings, being coherent, unpredictable variation over course of day) 0. No 1. Yes
		b. In the last 90 days (or since last assessment if less than 90 days), client has become agitated or disoriented such that his or her safety is endangered or client requires protection by others 0. No 1. Yes

SECTION C. COMMUNICATION/HEARING PATTERNS

1.	HEARING	*(With hearing appliance if used)* 0. HEARS ADEQUATELY—normal talk, TV, phone, doorbell 1. MINIMAL DIFFICULTY when not in quiet setting 2. HEARS IN SPECIAL SITUATIONS ONLY—speaker has to adjust tonal quality and speak distinctly 3. HIGHLY IMPAIRED — absence of useful hearing
2.	MAKING SELF UNDER-STOOD	*(Expressing information content—however able)* 0. UNDERSTOOD 1. USUALLY UNDERSTOOD—difficulty finding words or finishing thoughts 2. SOMETIMES UNDERSTOOD—ability is limited to making concrete requests 3. RARELY/NEVER UNDERSTOOD
3.	ABILITY TO UNDER-STAND OTHERS	*(Understands verbal information—however able)* 0. UNDERSTANDS 1. USUALLY UNDERSTANDS—may miss some part/intent of message 2. SOMETIMES UNDERSTANDS—responds adequately to simple, direct communication 3. RARELY/NEVER UNDERSTANDS

SECTION D. VISION PATTERNS

1.	VISION	*(Ability to see in adequate light and with glasses if used)* 0. ADEQUATE—sees fine detail, including regular print in newspapers/books 1. IMPAIRED—sees large print, but not regular print in newspapers/books 2. MODERATELY IMPAIRED—limited vision; not able to see newspaper headlines, but can identify objects 3. HIGHLY IMPAIRED—object identification in question, but eyes appear to follow objects 4. SEVERELY IMPAIRED—no vision or sees only light, colors, or shapes; eyes do not appear to follow objects
2.	VISUAL LIMITATION/DIFFICULTIES	Saw halos or rings around lights, curtains over eyes, or flashes of lights 0. No 1. Yes
3.	VISION DECLINE	Worsening of vision as compared to status of 90 days ago (or since last assessment if less than 90 days) 0. No 1. Yes

SECTION E. MOOD AND BEHAVIOR PATTERNS

1.	INDICATORS OF DEPRES-SION, ANXIETY, SAD MOOD	*(Code for indicators observed in last 30 days (or since last assessment if less than 30 days), irrespective of the assumed cause)* 0. Indicator not exhibited in last 30 days 1. Indicator of this type exhibited up to five days a week 2. Indicator of this type exhibited daily or almost daily (6, 7 days a week)

a. A feeling of sadness or being depressed, that life is not worth living, that nothing matters, that he or she is of no use to anyone or would rather be dead	e. Repetitive anxious complaints, concerns—e.g., persistently seeks attention/reassurance regarding schedules, meals, laundry, clothing, relationship issues
b. Persistent anger with self or others—e.g., easily annoyed, anger at care received	f. Sad, pained, worried facial expressions — e.g., furrowed brows
c. Expressions of what appear to be unrealistic fears—e.g., fear of being abandoned, left alone, being with others	g. Recurrent crying, tearfulness
d. Repetitive health complaints—e.g., persistently seeks medical attention, obsessive concern with body functions	h. Withdrawal from activities of interest—e.g., no interest in long standing activities or being with family/friends
	i. Reduced social interaction

2.	BEHAVIORAL SYMPTOMS	In the last 7 days, instances when the client exhibited following behavioral symptoms. If EXHIBITED, ease of altering the symptom when it occurred. 0. Did not occur in last 7 days 1. Occurred, easily altered 2. Occurred, not easily altered	
		a. WANDERING (moved with no rational purpose, seemingly oblivious to needs or safety)	
		b. VERBALLY ABUSIVE BEHAVIORAL SYMPTOMS (threatened, screamed at, cursed at others)	
		c. PHYSICALLY ABUSIVE BEHAVIORAL SYMPTOMS (hit, shoved, scratched, sexually abused others)	
		d. SOCIALLY INAPPROPRIATE/DISRUPTIVE BEHAVIORAL SYMPTOMS (disruptive sounds, noisiness, screaming, self-abusive acts, sexual behavior or disrobing in public, smears/throws food/ feces, rummaging, repetitive behavior, rises early and causes disruption)	
		e. AGGRESSIVE RESISTANCE OF CARE (e.g., threw medications, pushed caregiver)	
3.	CHANGES IN BEHAVIOR SYMPTOMS	Behavioral symptoms have become worse or are less well tolerated by family as compared to 30 days ago (or since last assessment if less than 30 days) 0. No, or no change in behavioral symptoms 1. Yes	

SECTION F. SOCIAL FUNCTIONING

1.	INVOLVE-MENT	a. Client is at ease interacting with others (e.g., likes to spend time with others) 0. At ease 1. Not at ease	
		b. Openly expresses conflict or anger with family/friends 0. No 1. Yes	
2.	CHANGE IN SOCIAL ACTIVITIES	As compared to 180 days ago (or since last assessment if less than 180 days ago), decline in the client's level of participation in social, religious, occupational or other preferred activities. IF THERE WAS A DECLINE, Client distressed by this fact 0. No decline 1. Decline, not distressed 2. Decline, distressed	
3.	ISOLATION	a. Length of time client is alone during the day (morning and afternoon) 0. Never or hardly ever 1. About one hour 2. Long periods of time—e.g., all morning 3. All of the time	
		b. Client says or indicates that he/she feels lonely 0. No 1. Yes	

SECTION G. INFORMAL SUPPORT SERVICES

1.	TWO KEY INFORMAL HELPERS Primary (A) and Secondary (B)	NAME OF PRIMARY AND SECONDARY HELPERS		
		a. (Last/Family Name) b. (First)		
		c. (Last/Family Name) d. (First)		
			(A) Prim	(B) Secn
		e. Lives with client 0. Yes 1. No 2. No such helper [skip other items]		
		f. Relationship to client 0. Child or child-in-law 2. Other Relative 1. Spouse 3. Friend/neighbor		
		Areas of help: 0. Yes 1. No		
		g. — Advice or emotional support		
		h. — IADL care		
		i. — ADL care		
		If needed, willingness (with ability) to increase help: 0. More than 2 hours 1. 1-2 hours per day 2. No		
		j. — Emotional support		
		k. — IADL care		
		l. — ADL care		
2.	CAREGIVER STATUS	(Check all that apply)	
		A caregiver is unable to continue in caring activities—e.g., decline in the health of the caregiver makes it difficult to continue	a.
		Primary caregiver is not satisfied with support received from family and friends (e.g., other children of client)	b.
		Primary caregiver expresses feelings of distress, anger or depression	c.
		NONE OF ABOVE	d.
3.	EXTENT OF HELP (HOURS OF CARE, ROUNDED)	For instrumental and personal activities of daily living received over the last 7 days, indicate extent of help from family, friends, and neighbors	HOURS
		a. Sum of time across five weekdays	
		b. Sum of time across two weekend days	

SECTION H. PHYSICAL FUNCTIONING (SELF PERFORMANCE OF INSTRUMENTAL (IADL) AND PERSONAL (ADL) ACTIVITIES OF DAILY LIVING)

1.	IADL SELF PERFORMANCE—Code for functioning in routine activities around the home or in the community during the last 7 days.		
	(A) IADL SELF PERFORMANCE CODE—(Code for client's performance during last 7 days) 0. INDEPENDENT—did on own 1. SOME HELP—help some of the time 2. FULL HELP—performed with help all of the time 3. BY OTHERS—performed by others 8. ACTIVITY DID NOT OCCUR		
	(B) IADL DIFFICULTY CODE How difficult it is (or would it be) for client to do activity on own 0. NO DIFFICULTY 1. SOME DIFFICULTY—e.g., needs some help, is very slow, or fatigues 2. GREAT DIFFICULTY—e.g., little or no involvement in the activity is possible	(A) Performance	(B) Difficulty

			(A)	(B)
a.	MEAL PREP-ARATION	How meals are prepared (e.g., planning meals, cooking, assembling ingredients, setting out food and utensils)		
b.	ORDINARY HOUSE WORK	How ordinary work around the house is performed (e.g., doing dishes, dusting, making bed, tidying up, laundry)		
c.	MANAGING FINANCE	How bills are paid, checkbook is balanced, household expenses are balanced		
d.	MANAGING MEDICA-TIONS	How medications are managed (e.g., remembering to take medicines, opening bottles, taking correct drug dosages, giving injections, applying ointments)		
e.	PHONE USE	How telephone calls are made or received (with assistive devices such as large numbers on telephone, amplification as needed)		
f.	SHOPPING	How shopping is performed for food and household items (e.g., selecting items, managing money)		
g.	TRANSPOR-TATION	How client travels by vehicle—e.g., gets to places beyond walking distance		

2.	ADL SELF-PERFORMANCE—The following address the client's physical functioning in routine personal activities of daily life, for example, dressing, eating, etc. during the last 7 days, considering all episodes of these activities. For clients who performed an activity independently, be sure to determine and record whether others encouraged the activity or were present to supervise or oversee the activity
0.	INDEPENDENT—No help or oversight —OR— Help/oversight provided only 1 or 2 times during last 7 days
1.	SUPERVISION—Oversight, encouragement or cueing provided 3 or more times during last 7 days —OR— Supervision (3 or more times) plus physical assistance provided only 1 or 2 times during last 7 days
2.	LIMITED ASSISTANCE—Client highly involved in activity; received physical help in guided maneuvering of limbs or other non-weight bearing assistance 3 or more times
3.	EXTENSIVE ASSISTANCE—While elder performed part of activity, over last 7-day period, help of following type(s) were provided 3 or more times: — Weight-bearing support —OR— — Full performance by another during part (but not all) of last 7 days
4.	TOTAL DEPENDENCE—Full performance of activity by another during entire 7 days
8.	ACTIVITY DID NOT OCCUR during entire 7 days (regardless of ability)

a.	MOBILITY IN BED	Including moving to and from lying position, turning side to side, and positioning body while in bed.		
b.	TRANSFER	Including moving to and between surfaces—to/from bed, chair, wheelchair, standing position. [Note—Excludes to/from bath/toilet]		
c.	LOCOMO-TION IN HOME	[Note—if in wheelchair, self-sufficiency once in chair]		
d.	DRESSING	Including laying out clothes, retrieving clothes from closet, putting clothes on and taking clothes off.		
e.	EATING	Including taking in food by any method, including tube feedings.		
f.	TOILET USE	Including using the toilet room or commode, bedpan, urinal, transferring on/off toilet, cleaning self after toilet use, changing pad, managing any special devices required (ostomy or catheter), and adjusting clothes.		
g.	PERSONAL HYGIENE	Including combing hair, brushing teeth, shaving, applying makeup, washing/drying face and hands, and perineum (EXCLUDE baths and showers).		
3.	BATHING	In the last 7 days (include shower, full tub or sponge bath; exclude washing back or hair) 0. INDEPENDENT, did on own 1. SUPERVISION— oversight help only 2. RECEIVED ASSISTANCE IN TRANSFER ONLY 3. RECEIVED ASSISTANCE IN PART OF BATHING ACTIVITY 4. TOTAL DEPENDENCE 8. ACTIVITY DID NOT OCCUR		
4.	PRIMARY MODES OF LOCOMO-TION	0. No assistive device 1. Cane 2. Walker/crutch 3. Scooter (e.g., Amigo) 4. Wheelchair 5. Activity does not occur		
		a. Indoors		
		b. Outdoors		

MDS-HC Draft 10a — 05/09/97

5.	STAIR CLIMBING	In the last 7 days, how client went up and down stairs (e.g., single or multiple steps, using handrail as needed). If client did not go up and down stairs, code client's capacity for stair climbing. 0. Up and down stairs without help 1. Up and down stairs with help 2. Not go up and down stairs—could do without help 3. Not go up and down stairs—could do with help 4. Not go up and down stairs—no capacity to do it 8. UNKNOWN—did not climb stairs and assessor is unable to judge whether the capacity exists	
6.	STAMINA	a. In a typical week, during the last 30 days, code the number of days client usually went out of the house or building in which client lives (no matter for how short a time period) 0. Every day 2. 1 day a week 1. 2-6 days a week 3. No days	
		b. Hours of physical activities in the last 7 days (e.g., walking, cleaning house, exercise) 0. Two or more hours 1. Less than two hours	
7.	FUNCTIONAL POTENTIAL	Client believes he/she capable of increased functional independence (ADL, IADL, mobility)	a.
		Caregivers believe client is capable of increased functional independence (ADL, IADL, mobility)	b.
		Good prospects of recovery from current disease or conditions, improved health status expected	c.
		NONE OF ABOVE	d.

SECTION L. CONTINENCE IN LAST 14 DAYS

1.	BLADDER CONTI-NENCE	In last 14 days (or since last assessment if less than 14 days) control of urinary bladder function (with appliances such as catheters or incontinence program employed) [Note—if dribbles, volume insufficient to soak through underpants] 0. CONTINENT—Complete control 1. USUALLY CONTINENT—Incontinent episodes once a week or less 2. OCCASIONALLY INCONTINENT—Incontinent episodes 2 or more times a week but not daily 3. FREQUENTLY INCONTINENT—Tends to be incontinent daily, but some control present 4. INCONTINENT—Inadequate control, multiple daily episodes	
2.	BLADDER DEVICES	(Check all that apply in last 14 days—or since last assessment if less than 14 days)	
		Use of pads or briefs to protect against wetness	a.
		Use of an indwelling urinary catheter	b.
		NONE OF ABOVE	c.
3.	BOWEL CONTI-NENCE	In last 14 days (or since last assessment if less than 14 days), control of bowel movement (with appliance or bowel continence program if employed) 0. CONTINENT—Complete control 1. USUALLY CONTINENT—Bowel incontinent episodes less than weekly 2. OCCASIONALLY INCONTINENT—Bowel incontinent episode once a week 3. FREQUENTLY INCONTINENT—Bowel incontinent episodes 2-3 times a week 4. INCONTINENT—Bowel incontinent all (or almost all) of the time	

SECTION J. DISEASE DIAGNOSES

Disease/infection that doctor has indicated is present and affects client's status, requires treatments, or requires symptom management. Also include if disease is being monitored by a health professional or is the reason for a hospitalization in last 90 days (or since last assessment if less than 90 days)
0. Not present
1. Present—not subject to focused treatment or monitoring by home care nurse
2. Present—monitored or treated by home care nurse

1.	DISEASES	HEART/CIRCULATION		o. Osteoporosis	
		a. Cerebrovascular accident (stroke)		SENSES	
		b. Congestive heart failure		p. Cataract	
		c. Coronary artery disease		q. Glaucoma	
		d. Hypertension		PSYCHIATRIC/MOOD	
		e. Irregularly irregular pulse		r. Any psychiatric diagnosis	
		f. Peripheral vascular disease		INFECTIONS	
		NEUROLOGICAL		s. HIV infection	
		g. Alzheimer's		t. Pneumonia	
		h. Dementia other than Alzheimer's disease		u. Tuberculosis	
		i. Head trauma		v. Urinary tract infection (in last 30 days)	
		j. Multiple sclerosis		OTHER DISEASES	
		k. Parkinsonism		w. Cancer—(in past 5 years) not including skin cancer	
		MUSCULO-SKELETAL		x. Diabetes	
		l. Arthritis		y. Emphysema/COPD/asthma	
		m. Hip fracture		z. Renal Failure	
		n. Other fractures (e.g., wrist, vertebra)		aa. Thyroid disease (hyper or hypo)	

2.	OTHER CURRENT OR MORE DETAILED DIAGNOSES AND ICD-9 CODES	a. _____					.		
		b. _____					.		
		c. _____					.		
		d. _____					.		

SECTION K. HEALTH CONDITIONS AND PREVENTIVE HEALTH MEASURES

1.	PREVENTIVE HEALTH	(Check all that apply—in past 2 years)	
		Blood pressure measured	a.
		Received influenza vaccination	b.
		IF FEMALE: Received breast examination or mammography	c.
		NONE OF ABOVE	d.

2.	PROBLEM CONDITIONS PRESENT ON 2 OR MORE DAYS	(Check all that were present on at least 2 of the last 7 days)			
		Diarrhea		Loss of appetite	d.
		Difficulty urinating or urinating 3 or more times at night	a.	Vomiting	e.
		Fever	b.	NONE OF ABOVE	f.

3.	PROBLEM CONDITIONS IN LAST WEEK	(Check all present at any point during last 7 days)			
		PHYSICAL HEALTH		Edema	e.
		Change in sputum production	a.	Shortness of breath	f.
		Chest pain at exertion or chest pain/pressure at rest	b.	MENTAL HEALTH	
				Delusions	g.
		Constipation in 4 of last 7 days	c.	Hallucinations	h.
		Dizziness or lightheadedness	d.	NONE OF ABOVE	i.

4.	PAIN	a. Frequently complains or shows evidence of pain (in last 7 days) 0. No pain 1. Pain less than daily 2. Pain daily (skip to item K4e)	
		b. Pain is unusually intense 0. No 1. Yes	
		c. Pain intensity disrupts usual activities 0. No 1. Yes	
		d. Character of pain 0. No pain 1. Localized - single site 2. Multiple sites	
		e. Pain controlled by medication 0. No pain 1. Medication offered no control 2. Pain is partially or fully controlled by medication	
5.	FALLS FREQUENCY	Number of times fell in last 180 days (or since last assessment if less than 180 days) If none, code "0"; if more than 9, code "9"	
6.	DANGER OF FALL	a. Unsteady gait 0. No 1. Yes	
		b. Client limits going outdoors due to fear of falling (e.g., stopped using bus, goes out only with others) 0. No 1. Yes	
7.	LIFE STYLE (Drinking/ Smoking)	a. In the last 90 days (or since last assessment if less than 90 days), client felt the need or was told by others to cut down on drinking, or others were concerned with client's drinking 0. No 1. Yes	
		b. In the last 90 days (or since last assessment if less than 90 days), client had to have a drink first thing in the morning to steady nerves (i.e., an "eye opener") or has been in trouble because of drinking 0. No 1. Yes	
		c. Over a typical week in the last month, record the number of days (0-7) client had one or more drinks	
		d. On days client had a drink, record the number of drinks usually consumed per day (code 0 for no drinks, 9 for 9 or more drinks)	
		e. Smoked or chewed tobacco daily 0. No 1. Yes	
8.	HEALTH STATUS INDICATORS	Client feels he/she has poor health (when asked)	a.
		Has conditions or diseases that make cognition, ADL, mood, or behavior patterns unstable (fluctuations, precarious, or deteriorating)	b.
		Experiencing a flare-up of a recurrent or chronic problem	c.
		Treatments changed in last 30 days (or since last assessment if less than 30 days) because of a new acute episode or condition	d.
		Prognosis of less than six months to live—e.g., physician has told client or client's family that client has end-stage disease	e.
		NONE OF ABOVE	f.
9.	OTHER STATUS INDICATORS	Fearful of a family member or caregiver	a.
		Unusually poor hygiene	b.
		Unexplained injuries, broken bones, or burns	c.
		Neglected, abused, or mistreated	d.
		Physically restrained (e.g., limbs restrained, used bed rails, constrained to chair when sitting)	e.
		NONE OF ABOVE	f.

SECTION L. NUTRITION/HYDRATION STATUS

1.	WEIGHT CHANGE	Unintended weight loss of 5% or more in the last 30 days or 10% or more in the last 180 days 0. No 1. Yes	
2.	CONSUMP- TION	a. In at least 4 of the last 7 days, ate one or fewer meals a day 0. No 1. Yes	
		b. In last 3 days, noticeable decrease in the amount of food client usually eats usually consumes 0. No 1. Yes	
		c. Insufficient fluid—did not consume all/almost all fluids during last 3 days 0. No 1. Yes	
3.	NUTRI- TIONAL- TREAT- MENTS	Number of days formal care received in last week	
		a. Intravenous or infusion therapy—hydration (not including TPN)	
		b. Fluids by mouth	
		c. Parenteral nutrition (TPN or lipids)	
		d. Enteral—tube feeding	

SECTION M. DENTAL STATUS (ORAL HEALTH)

1.	ORAL STATUS	(Check all that apply)	
		Problem chewing or swallowing (e.g., pain while eating)	a.
		Mouth is "dry" when eating a meal	b.
		Problem brushing teeth or dentures	c.
		NONE OF ABOVE	d.

SECTION N. SKIN CONDITION

1.	SKIN PROBLEMS	Any troubling skin conditions or changes in the last 30 days (e.g., burns, bruises, rashes, itchiness, body lice, scabies) 0. No 1. Yes	
2.	ULCERS (Pressure/ Stasis)	Presence of an ulcer anywhere on the body. Ulcers include any area of persistent skin redness (Stage 1); partial loss of skin layers (Stage 2); deep craters in the skin (Stage 3); and breaks in skin exposing muscle or bone (Stage 4). [Code 0 if no ulcer, otherwise record the highest ulcer stage (Stage 1-4).]	
		a. Pressure ulcer—any lesion caused by pressure, shear forces, resulting in damage of underlying tissues	
		b. Stasis ulcer—open lesion caused by poor circulation in the lower extremities	
3.	OTHER SKIN PROBLEMS REQUIRING TREATMENT	(Check all that apply)	

	Surgical Wounds Sites	
Burns (second or third degree)	a.	Thorax	d.
Open lesions other than ulcers, rashes, cuts (e.g., cancer)	b.	Abdomen	e.
		Extremities	f.
Skin tears or cuts	c.	Other	g.
		NONE OF ABOVE	h.

4.	HISTORY OF RESOLVED PRESSURE ULCERS	Client previously had (at any time) or has an ulcer anywhere on the body 0. No 1. Yes	
5.	WOUND/ ULCER CARE	Number of days formal care received in last week	
		a. Antibiotics, systemic or topical	
		b. Dressings	
		c. Pressure reduction/relieving devices	
		d. Nutrition or hydration	
		e. Turning/repositioning	
		f. Debridement	
		g. Surgical wound care	
6.	FOOT PROBLEMS	(Check all that apply)	
		Corns, calluses, structural problems, infections, fungi	a.
		Open lesions on the foot	b.
		Foot not inspected in last 90 days by client or other	c.
		NONE OF ABOVE	d.

SECTION O. ENVIRONMENTAL ASSESSMENT

1.	HOME ENVIRON- MENT (Check any of following that make home environment hazardous or uninhabit- able (If none apply, check NONE OF ABOVE.) If temporarily in institution, base assessment on home visit)]	Lighting in evening (including inadequate or no lighting in living room, sleeping room kitchen, toilet, corridors)	a.
		Flooring and carpeting (e.g., holes in floor, electric wires where client walks, scatter rugs)	b.
		Bathroom and toiletroom (e.g., non-operating toilet, leaking pipes, no rails though needed, slippery bathtub, outside toilet)	c.
		Kitchen (e.g., dangerous stove, inoperative refrigerator, infestation by rats or bugs)	d.
		Heating and cooling (e.g., too hot in summer, too cold in winter, wood stove in a home with an asthmatic)	e.
		Personal safety (e.g., fear of violence, safety problem in going to mailbox or visiting neighbors, heavy traffic in street)	f.
		Access to home (e.g., difficulty entering/leaving home)	g.
		Access to rooms in house (e.g., unable to climb stairs)	h.
		NONE OF ABOVE	i.
2.	LIVING ARRANGE- MENT	a. As compared to 90 days ago, client now lives with other persons— e.g., moved in with another person, other moved in with client 0. No 1. Yes	
		b. Client or primary caregiver feels that client would be better off in another living environment 0. No 1. Client only 2. Caregiver only 3. Client and caregiver	

SECTION P. SERVICE UTILIZATION

1.	FORMAL CARE (Minutes rounded to even 10 minutes)	Extent of care or care management in last 14 days (or since last assessment if less than 14 days) involving		(A) # of Days	(B) Hours	(C) Mins
		a. Home health aides				
		b. Visiting nurses				
		c. Homemaking services				
		d. Meals				
		e. Volunteer services				
		f. Physical therapy				
		g. Occupational therapy				
		h. Speech therapy				
		i. Day care or day hospital				
		j. Social worker in home				

2.	SPECIAL TREAT- MENTS, THERAPIES, PROGRAMS	Special treatments, therapies, and programs received or scheduled during the last 14 days (or since last assessment if less than 14 days) and adherence to the required schedule. Includes services received in the home or on an outpatient basis. 0. Not applicable 1. Scheduled, full adherence as prescribed 2. Scheduled, partial adherence 3. Scheduled, not received

TREATMENTS		a. Ventilator	
a. Alcohol/drug treatment program		THERAPIES	
		t. Exercise therapy	
b. Blood transfusions		u. Occupational therapy	
c. Chemotherapy		v. Physical therapy	
d. Cardiac rehabilitation		w. Respiratory therapy (including suctioning, IPPB)	
e. Continuous positive airway pressure (CPAP)		PROGRAMS	
f. Dialysis-peritoneal (CAPD)		x. Day center	
g. Dialysis-renal		y. Day hospital	
h. Holter monitor		z. Hospice care	
i. IV infusion - central		aa. Physician or clinic visit	
j. IV infusion - peripheral		bb. Respite care	
k. Medication by injection		SPECIAL PROCEDURES DONE IN HOME	
l. Ostomy care			
m. Oxygen therapy - intermittent		cc. Daily nurse monitoring (e.g., EKG, urinary output)	
n. Oxygen therapy - continuous (concentrator)		dd. Nurse monitoring less than daily	
o. Oxygen therapy - continuous (other)		ee. Medical alert bracelet or electronic security alert	
p. Radiation therapy		ff. Skin treatment	
q. Respiratory therapy		gg. Special diet	
r. Tracheostomy care		hh. Other	

3.	MANAGE-MENT OF EQUIPMENT (In Last 14 Days)	Management codes: 0. Not used 1. Managed on own 2. Managed on own if laid out or with verbal reminders 3. Partially performed by others 4. Fully performed by others		
		a. Oxygen	c. Catheter	
		b. IV		
4.	VISITS IN LAST 90 DAYS OR SINCE LAST ASSESS-MENT	*Enter 0 if none, if more than 9, code "9"*		
		a. Number of times ADMITTED TO HOSPITAL with an overnight stay		
		b. Number of times VISITED EMERGENCY ROOM without an overnight stay		
		c. EMERGENT CARE—including unscheduled nursing, physician, or theraputic visits to office or home		
5.	TREATMENT GOALS	Any treatment goals that have been met in the last 90 days (or since last assessment if less than 90 days)? 0. No 1. Yes		
6.	OVERALL CHANGE IN CARE NEEDS	Overall self sufficiency has changed significantly as compared to status of 90 days ago (or since last assessment if less than 90 days) 0. No change 1. Improved—receives fewer 2. Deteriorated—receives supports more support		
7.	TRADE OFFS	Because of limited funds, during the last month, client made trade-offs among purchasing any of the following: prescribed medications, sufficient home heat, necessary physician care, adequate food, home care 0. No 1. Yes		

SECTION Q. MEDICATIONS

1.	NUMBER OF MEDICA-TIONS	Record the number of different medicines (prescriptions and over the counter), including eye drops, taken regularly or on an occasional basis in the last 7 days [*If none, code "0", if more than 8, code "9"*]		
2.	RECEIPT OF PSYCHO-TROPIC MEDICATION	Psychotropic medications taken in the last 7 days [Note—Review client's medications with the list that applies to the following categories] 0. No 1. Yes		
		a. Antipsychotic	c. Antidepressant	
		b. Antianxiety	d. Hypnotic	
3.	MEDICAL OVERSIGHT	Physician reviewed client's medications as a whole in last 180 days 0. Discussed with at least one physician (or no medication taken) 1. No single physician reviewed all medications		
4.	COMPLI-ANCE/ ADHERENCE WITH MEDICA-TIONS	Compliant all or most of time with medications prescribed by physician (both during and between therapy visits) 0. Always compliant 1. Compliant 80% of time or more 2. Compliant less than 80% of time 3. *NO MEDICATIONS PRESCRIBED*		

5.	LIST OF ALL MEDICA-TIONS	List prescribed and nonprescribed medications taken in last 7 days
		a. Name and Dose—Record the name of the medication and dose ordered.
		b. Form: Code the route of Administration using the following list:
		   1=by mouth (PO) 5=subcutaneous (SQ) 8=inhalation
		   2=sub lingual (SL) 6=rectal (R) 9=enteral tube
		   3=intramuscular (IM) 7=topical 10=other
		   4=intravenous (IV)		

d. Freq: Code the number of times per day, week, or month the medication is administered using the following list:

PR=(PRN) as necessary	2D=(BID) two times daily	QO=every other day
1H=(QH) every hour	(includes every 12 hrs)	4W=4 times each week
2H=(Q2H) every two hours	3D=(TID) three times daily	5W=five times each week
3H=(Q3H) every three hours	4D=(QID) four times daily	6W=six times each week
4H=(Q4H) every four hours	5D=five times daily	1M=(Q month) once every month
6H=(Q6H) every six hours	1W=(Q week) once each wk	2M=twice every month
8H=(Q8H) every eight hours	2W=two times every week	C=continuous
1D=(QD or HS) once daily	3W=three times every week	O=other

a. Name and Dose	b. Form	c. Number Taken	d. Freq.
a. _____			
b. _____			
c. _____			
d. _____			
e. _____			
f. _____			
g. _____			
h. _____			
i. _____			
j. _____			
k. _____			

Appendix 2

Client Assessment Protocol — Falls

Objective

To ascertain if falls have occurred recently and if the client is at risk of falling, and to provide care planning guidance for minimizing the risk of falls and limiting the extent of possible injury.

Triggers

Potential for additional falls or risk of initial fall suggested if one or more of following present:

- Dizziness or lightheadedness in last seven days [K3d = checked]
- Falls frequency. Number of falls in the last 180 days [K5=1 or more]
- Has unsteady (abnormal) gait [K6a=1]
- Limits going outdoors due to fear of falling [K6b=1]
- More than 6 medications [Q1=7 or more]
- Antipsychotic medication [Q2a=1]
- Antianxiety medication [Q2b=1]
- Antidepressant medication [Q2c=1]

Definition

Fall: An unintentional change in position where the elder ends up on the floor or ground. A fall may result from intrinsic or extrinsic causes or both. Falls represent an important geriatric syndrome, not only because of their prevalence, morbidity and mortality, but also because they can be the 'tip of the iceberg' of significant but unrecognized underlying illness. Falls provide an opportunity to identify undiagnosed illnesses and disabilities which when addressed may halt imminent functional decline.

Background

Each year, one third of the elderly living in the community fall, with about half falling more than once. The risk of falls increases with age, as does morbidity and mortality. Up to 5 per cent of falls result in fractures, of which one of the most serious is of the hip. Significant soft tissue injuries occur in about 10 per cent of falls.

Fear is an important consequence of falls, commonly resulting in a curtailing of activities. Fear of falling is reported as characteristic of 40 per cent or more of those who fall, while 41 per cent of those persons can be expected to experience a restriction in activity over the ensuing 6-month period.

In some instances a single causal factor can explain the fall, more frequently multiple factors can be identified. Many chronic conditions serve as a 'substrate' for falls with the fall occurring when the environment poses a hazard or an acute illness sets in.

Five major 'intrinsic' risk-factor categories for falls

1 *Neuromuscular risk factors.* Gait disorders (e.g., those seen in Parkinson's disease, multi-infarct dementia and both focal and generalized muscle weakness).
2 *Cardiovascular risk factors.* Postural, postprandial, and drug-induced hypotension. [Note, Syncope can be considered a special case of falls].
3 *Orthopedic risk factors.* Skeletal pain and deformities, podiatric difficulties, leg-length discrepancy, and a displaced center of gravity secondary to orthopedic disease, fractures, or arthritis.
4 *Perceptual risk factors.* Various combinations of visual and labyrinthine deficits as well as impaired position sense.
5 *Psychiatric and behavioral disorders.* Depression, delirium and dementia which can cause poor judgment leading to unsafe behaviour.

Three 'extrinsic' risk factors for falls

1 *Medications.* Sedatives, neuroleptics, antidepressants and cardiovascular medications which produce hypotension, extrapyramidal effects, or a decreased level of alertness.
2 *Alcohol use.* Not only the alcoholic intoxication but the disabilities, such as peripheral neuropathy, associated with chronic excessive alcohol consumption.
3 *Various environmental hazards.* Poor illumination, throw rugs, patterned carpets, stairways, slippery floors, and uneven surfaces (see Environmental CAP).

Guidelines

Problem review

For those who have fallen, review relevant information on the fall and refer to a physician for detailed work up. Review the circumstances under which the fall occurred.

- Was the activity usual or unusual?
- Was the environment usual or unusual?
- What time of day did it occur?
- Were there any symptoms at the time, such as urinary urgency or light headedness?
- What does the elder see as a logical preventive measure?
- Did it occur from a standing or sitting position?
- How does the elder assess the fall?

For all who have been triggered including those who have not fallen, complete the following evaluation to identify intrinsic and extrinsic risk factors, as well as any induced fear of falling. Many of the procedures will require referral to the physician. Appropriate safety precautions are essential among the elderly and the individual should be thoroughly evaluated first by a physician if there is any indication of a significant injury such as a fracture, concussion, or serious soft tissue injury from a fall which has already occurred.

Review of intrinsic factors

Cardiovascular evaluation.
- (Nurse evaluators) Measure blood pressure lying and standing, at one and three minutes. Is there a postural systolic blood pressure reduction of 20 mm Hg or greater or a blood pressure level below 90 mm Hg standing.
- Was there a sudden loss of consciousness or nearly so (syncope)?

Neuromuscular evaluation.
- (Nurse evaluators) Modifications will be necessary if assistive devices are required. Check for a focal weakness, increased tone, or loss of position sense. It is valuable to observe the elder's gait and balance and, if appropriate, to observe the elder perform the activity that may have led to a fall.
- Are there new or worsening chest symptoms, such as chest pain or shortness of breath? Refer to a physician if any of the abnormalities are found.
- Have the person stand up from a chair with crossed arms at the chest, if possible. Inability to do this may be a sign of leg muscle weakness and a risk factor for falls.
- Observe the elder's gait for characteristics of initiation, speed, step-height, step-length, step-symmetry, and arm swing. Watch the person increase and reduce gait speed. Can the individual walk a straight path?
- Watch for difficulties with balance while sitting, standing up from a chair, and turning.
- Observe the person standing with legs together and eyes open and closed. Give the person a light nudge on the chest and observe the response. Extra special attention to safety should be taken.
- Observe the elder stand on one leg or walk a line.

Make a note of difficulties and see tables at end of this CAP for possible solutions.

Special senses. For vision impairment, see CAP on Vision.
- Question the elder as to the presence of dizziness or a sensation of loss of balance and if present, the circumstances of its occurrence.

Cognitive evaluation. See CAP on Cognition.

Mood evaluation. See CAP on Depression.

Evaluation for need for assistive devices. See CAP on ADLs.

Evaluation for the presence of acute illness. If any signs or symptoms of an acute illness are present, appropriate medical referral is indicated.

Review of extrinsic factors

Medications. A complete review of medications should be undertaken in consultation with a physician with the goal of simplifying the regimen, eliminating drugs no longer needed and prescribing to lowest effective dose of each drug. In addition, each medication should be assessed to determine if it may have contributed to a fall or risk of falling. (See CAP on Medication Management).

Alcohol. See Alcohol CAP.

Environmental hazards. See Environmental Assessment CAP and table at the end of this CAP. Assess the environment with specific reference to the unique disabilities of the individual being screened.

Since multiple factors may contribute to a fall, often in a summative manner, each intrinsic and extrinsic factor identified should be modified to the extent possible. Several principles of rehabilitation with special focus to strengthening of the lower extremities and improving balance may be exceedingly valuable. Physical therapy referrals for advice as to the availability of assistive devices may be useful. Ophthalmologic referral is indicated for visually impaired clients who have not been so evaluated in the recent past.

See Tables at the end of this CAP for further guidance.

Table A.2.1. Intrinsic risk factors for falling and possible interventions

Risk factor	Range of possible interventions	
	Medical	Rehabilitative or environmental
Reduced visual acuity and dark adaption	Eye examination; refraction, cataract extraction	Home safety assessment
Vestibular dysfunction (dizziness)	Avoidance of drugs affecting the vestibular system; neurologic or ear, nose, and throat evaluation, if indicated	Balance exercises
Proprioceptive dysfunction, cervical degenerative disorders, and peripheral neuropathy	Screening for vitamin B_{12} deficiency and cervical spondylosis	Balance exercises; appropriate walking aid; correctly sized footwear with firm soles; home safety assessment
Dementia	Detection of reversible causes; avoidance of sedative or centrally acting drugs	Supervised exercise and ambulation; home safety assessment
Musculoskeletal disorders	Appropriate diagnostic evaluation	Balance-and-gait training; muscle-strengthening exercises; appropriate walking aid; home safety assessment
Foot disorders (calluses, bunion, deformities)	Shaving of calluses; bunionectomy	Trimming of nails; appropriate footwear
Postural hypotension	Assessment of medications; rehydration; possible alteration in situational factors (e.g., meals, change of position)	Dorsiflexion exercises; pressure-graded stockings; elevation of head of bed
Use of medications (sedatives: benzodiazepines, phenothiazines; antidepressants; antihypertensives; others: antiarrhythmics, anticonvulsants, diuretics, alcohol)	Steps to be taken: 1. Attempted reduction in the total no. of medications taken 2. Assessment of risks and benefits of each medication 3. Selection of medication, if needed, that is least centrally acting, least associated with postural hypotension, and has shortest action 4. Prescription of lowest effective dose 5. Frequent reassessment of risks and benefits	

Table A.2.2. Elements in the assessment of balance and gait

Abnormality	Possible diagnoses	Rehabilitative or environmental interventions
BALANCE		
Difficulty in getting up from and sitting down in chair	Myopathy; arthritis; Parkinson's syndrome; postural hypotension; deconditioning	Exercises to strengthen lower extremities; transfer training; high firm chairs with arms; raised toilet seats
Unsteadiness during neck turning and extension	Cervical degenerative disorder (e.g., arthritis, spondylosis)	Neck exercises; cervical collar; appropriate storage of items in kitchen and bedroom
Unsteadiness after nudge on sternum	Parkinson's syndrome; normal pressure hydrocephalus; other central nervous system disease; back problems	Balance training; back exercises; obstacle-free environment; appropriate walking aid; night light
GAIT		
Decreased step height	Central nervous system disease; multiple sensory deficits (visual, vestibular, proprioceptive); fear of falling	Careful sensory evaluation; gait training; proper footwear; appropriate walking aid; low pile carpet or nonskid floor without throw rugs
Unsteadiness on uneven surfaces	Decreased proprioception; ankle weakness; balance disorders	Gait training; appropriate footwear; appropriate walking aid; avoidance of thick carpet
Unsteadiness while turning	Parkinson's syndrome; multiple sensory deficits; cerebellar disease; hemiparesis; loss of visual field	Gait training; proprioceptive exercises; appropriate walking aid; obstacle-free environment
Increased path deviation	Cerebellar disease; balance disorders; sensory or motor ataxia; multiple sensory deficits	Gait training; appropriate walking aid

Table A.2.3. Environmental factors affecting the risk of falling in the home

Environmental area or factor	Objective and recommendations
Lighting	Absence of glare and shadows; accessible switches at room entrances; night light in bedroom, hall, bathroom
Floors	Nonskid backing for throw rugs; carpet edges tacked down; carpets with shallow pile; nonskid wax on floors; cords out of walking path; small objects (e.g., clothes, shoes) off floor
Stairs	Lighting sufficient, with switches at top and bottom of stairs; securely fastened bilateral handrails that stand out from wall; top and bottom steps marked with bright, contrasting tape; stair rises of no more than 6 inches; steps in good repair; no objects stored on steps
Kitchen	Items stored so that reaching up and bending over are not necessary; secure step stool available if climbing is necessary; firm, nonmovable table
Bathroom	Grab bars for tub, shower, and toilet; nonskid decals or rubber mat in tub or shower; shower chair with hand-held shower; nonskid rugs; raised toilet seat; door locks removed to ensure access in an emergency
Yard and entrances	Repair of cracks in pavement, holes in lawn; removal of rocks, tools, and other tripping hazards; well-lit walkways, free of ice and wet leaves; stairs and steps as above
Institutions	All the above; bed at proper height (not too high or low); spills on floor cleaned up promptly; appropriate use of walking aids and wheelchairs
Footwear	Shoes with firm, nonskid, nonfriction soles; low heels (unless person is accustomed to high heels); avoidance of walking in stocking feet or loose slippers

AUTHORS
Palmi V. Jónsson, MD
Douglas P. Kiel, MD
Lewis A. Lipsitz, MD

Reproduced from Morris et al. (1997).

8 Social Services Departments, Secondary Health Care and Community Care

Peter Huxley

The terms primary, secondary and tertiary care might once have been useful for describing the structure of the health service, but they are inadequate for the description of modern community care practice. This is in part because the terms are used as if they distinguish structures, whereas they actually distinguish functions. People with long-term and complex needs require services which integrate health and social care assessments and care packages, often from each of the so-called primary, secondary and tertiary services. The integration of functions might take place horizontally (between health and social care) or vertically (upwards from task, case, professional to management and agency), and in both cases could be described as functional integration. Horizontal integration of functions at the case or task level requires integration or collaboration at the other system levels in order to be sustained. The Darlington Project suggests that both horizontal and vertical (functional) integration and collaboration are critical to the success of community care.

The essence of the primary/secondary distinction is that the patient/client goes first to certain places or agencies, and if these agents do not perform the required functions then they usually refer the client to someone who does. In health care this is likely to be a consultant who conducts further more detailed assessment. Following the assessment, care and/or treatment may be provided, but this agency will also refer on to another provider (who is the third or tertiary agent) if they are

unable to make a suitable provision to meet need. Social services departments also provide primary (front-line open access), secondary (assessment and care management) and sometimes tertiary care (specialist
residential provisions).

In addition, one can take it as axiomatic that primary health care is
not simply to be equated with general medical practice or practitioners.
Likewise, to identify secondary care with hospital services is to confuse
location with function. Not all hospital care is secondary. Some people
present themselves to accident and emergency services directly, but
also doctors employed by hospitals can encounter new patients in
various community settings.

Insofar as these systems do exist in both social services and health,
there is a massive potential for referral systems to produce discon-
tinuous, uncoordinated care. Figure 8.1 indicates that there are 32

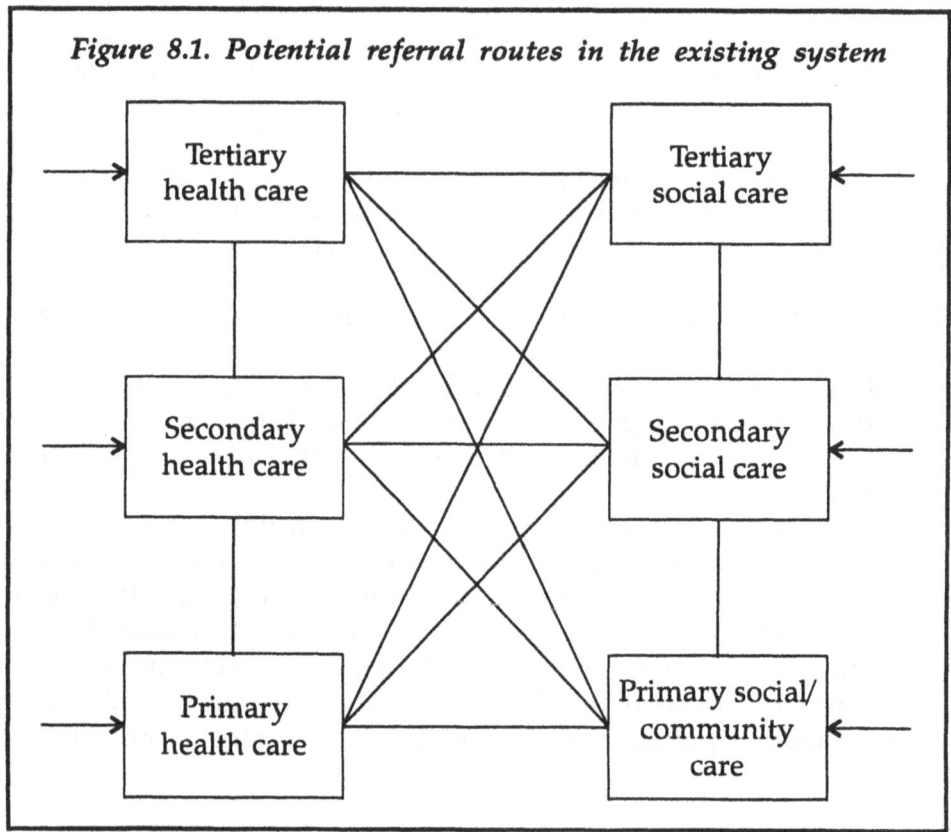

Figure 8.1. Potential referral routes in the existing system

pathways/referral mechanisms, with thirteen obvious filters. The ones coming straight in at the tertiary level come from other constituencies, such as the criminal justice system, for example.

The concepts of primary, secondary and tertiary care are therefore inadequate and misleading in many ways for people with complex health and social care needs. Such people usually require the combined services of both health and social care agencies, and may require packages of care from all the levels at once. Discharged forensic patients could be one example.

The current conception of the primary/secondary interface in use in the NHS Research and Development Initiative is not very useful because it tends to focus attention upon the health service structures which existed before the current reforms. Alternative concepts are needed which are more obviously related to the integration of health and social care needs, are independent of location, and are a more realistic reflection of the current mixed economy of welfare.

The Darlington model used by PSSRU is one example (Challis et al., 1995). This involved case-finding and screening for a predetermined target group, and the integration of care elements from different sources into a care package, together with the integration of what were previously discrete health and social services functions within the same worker. Another more functional model is that suggested by Max Marshall (personal communication). His model contains functional concepts of spotters, assessors and specialists. Spotters identify needs but are not equipped to assess complex needs and so refer cases to those who are (assessors). Assessors may not be able to provide long-term care for defined groups and so refer on to specialists who can do so. This differs from the primary/secondary distinction because it is more clearly based on function. One agency can provide different functions for different client groups, i.e. be a spotter for one but a specialist for another.

What the Darlington Project and similar experiments in the USA in mental health offer, is a service which does not operate according to the traditional divisions (in terms of agencies, locations and referral systems), but which offer instead a more integrated approach. It might be helpful at this point to distinguish between the concepts of integration and coordination:

- *coordination* is the harmonious combination of agents or functions towards the production of a result; and

- *integration* is the making up of a whole by adding together or combining the separate parts or elements.

One might make the distinction between vertical and horizontal integration, the latter being mainly of health and social care functions, while the former, rather than being concerned with the traditional structural terms (primary, secondary etc.) covers the agency/management/professional/case/task hierarchy outlined by Challis et al. (1995) and shown in Figure 8.2.

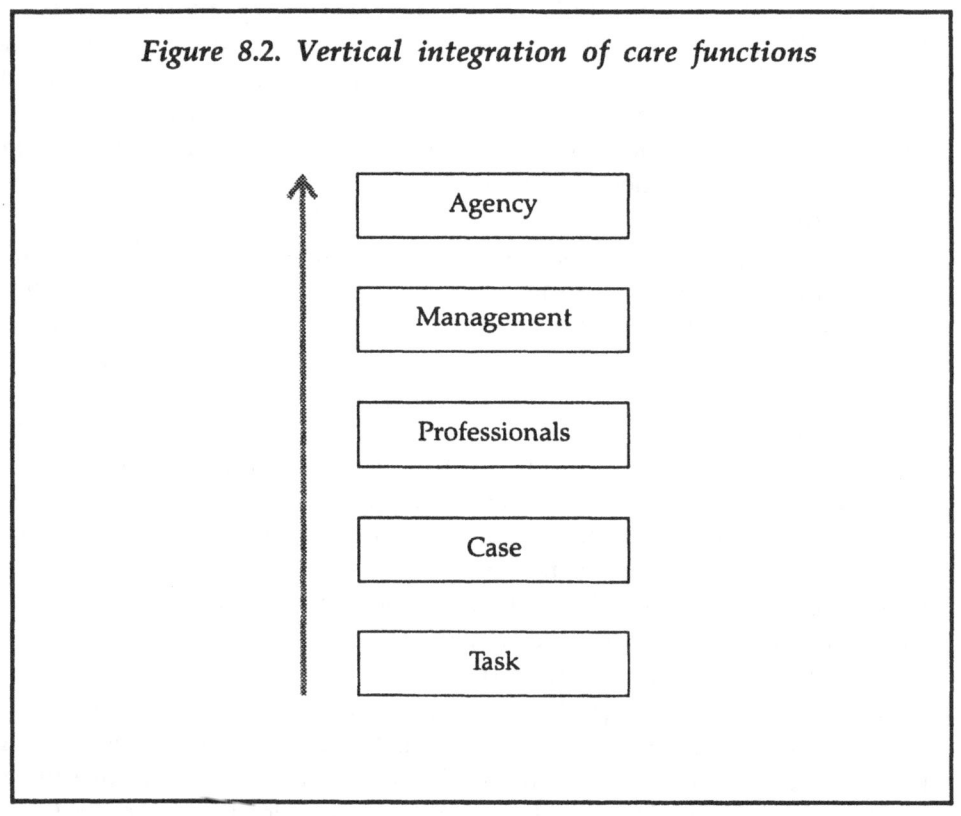

Figure 8.2. Vertical integration of care functions

The primary/secondary interface in mental health care

The work of Goldberg and Huxley on the primary/secondary care interface in mental health is relevant to disentangling these issues, and

Table 8.1. The Goldberg-Huxley model

Level 1 The community	
Filter 1 Illness/consulting behaviour	230[a]
Level 2 Primary care	
Filter 2 Recognition by family doctor	101
Level 3 Conspicuous disorder	
Filter 3 Decision by GP to refer	21
Level 4 Secondary care	
Filter 4 Decision to admit	3.4
Level 5 Admission	

a Figures are one year period prevalence per 1,000 population (community rate 250-315).

is therefore reviewed briefly here (Goldberg and Huxley, 1980, 1995). The central thesis of the model is that the patient has to pass a series of obstacles before arriving at specialist psychiatric care. They described these obstacles as filters between different levels of care. Each filter is 'selectively permeable', which means that some patients go through it more easily than others. There are four filters and five levels, as shown in Table 8.1.

It can be seen that the primary care physician plays a key role in the pathway to psychiatric care, and so the ways in which they recognise disorder and decide to deal with it are the most important filters.

The critical factor for our present purpose is the fact that, although the model is presented as if it were a structural model, based on the primary/secondary interface, it is in fact a process or functional model. Each of the filters is dependent upon decision-making processes about the type of needs presented and the package of care which is appropriate to meet these needs. The recognition of the problem or disorder is a function of the GP's assessment abilities, and the decision to refer to a specialist is based on the perceived difficulty of the assessment, or the difficulty of treatment, or the failure of prior attempts to meet the patient's identified needs.

In spite of much publicity, training programmes, and feedback to GPs, the performance of primary care in adequately assessing and treating patients with mental illness remains very much as it was in the late 1970s, when this model was quantified. A number of unrelated studies lend weight to this assertion. GPs continue to miss major depression, especially in cases where there is associated physical illness (Blacker and Clare, 1987); there is a low level of recognition by GPs of depression in those over 70 reported from Australia (Bowers et al., 1990); their diagnostic assessments are inferior to standardised instruments (Mari et al., 1987); they fail to recognise more than half of the psychological disorders which are presented to them as somatic complaints (Bridges and Goldberg, 1992); and they are more likely to refer patients on to a psychiatrist if the patient has attendant social difficulties (Giel et al., 1990).

In the UK the original work was seized upon by those for whom there was an advantage in seeing most morbidity either as untreated in the community or largely the responsibility of GPs. To caricature these responses (only slightly), they were as follows. For GPs, their main conclusion was that they were treating most morbidity and therefore required more help from psychiatrists, and, latterly, for purchasers to give greater priority to the sort of cases they primarily treated. The model lent weight to an argument for closer association between psychiatrists and GPs, and many outreach and liaison schemes began as a consequence. Among social workers, many saw their departments as having greater responsibility because the bulk of disorder was in the community and psychiatrists only saw a small proportion of it. This contributed to their assuming that they, and not health, should have the lead responsibility. Public health doctors saw the problem as a public health issue, and also focused on the fact that the bulk of disorder is in the community or at primary care level. Many public health doctors take this as an indication that services should focus on prevention, particularly primary prevention. Psychiatrists, on the other hand, have focused on the permeability of the filters to severe disorders, and have become concerned that adequate resources are targeted upon the severely ill, and not dispersed into primary prevention, primary care, or social services. Politicians have seized upon the idea that hospital is not the primary location of care, and have tended to neglect the issue of serious illness. Finally, planners and politicians have attempted to reduce the number of hospital beds and refocus these services in community settings.

These fundamental misperceptions of the original model concern severe disorders. Severe, long-term, disabling and complex cases are:

(a) of low prevalence in community settings, especially at the level of the individual GP; (b) pass through the filters to secondary care much more quickly than common disorder; and (c) present coordination and control problems which are more easily resolved in a hospital but which are very difficult to overcome in the community.

A more integrated system requires that the filters become extremely permeable or disappear altogether, and that the social aspects of assessment and care are provided at the same time as clinical ones. This was not clearly stated in the structure of the original model (Goldberg and Huxley, 1980, 1992), although there was discussion about the central significance of social aspects in the causes, courses, treatments and outcomes of common and severe mental disorders. This takes us to the limitations of the primary health care model.

The limitations of the primary health care model in the mental health context

Those who keep on repeating the mantra 'GPs have a crucial role to play' appear to make erroneous assumptions about the GP's role. Kendrick's (1992) survey of 369 GPs in the old South West Thames Region found a depressing picture in respect of GPs' desires and attitudes to the care of long-term severely mentally ill people. Kendrick's findings were published in several places, one of them an HMSO publication on *The Primary Care of Schizophrenia* (1992). There are three different perceptions in this publication of the extent of the average GP's contact with people with severe and long-term mental illness. The first is Kendrick's, the second is that of the vice-chairman of the Royal College of General Practitioners (Davies, 1992), and the third is that of Strathdee, now with the Department of Health (Strathdee, 1992). Davies states that the average GP is likely to have only three chronic cases on their list. On this basis a GP would need a list size five times the average simply to achieve the equivalent of one intensive case manager's caseload. Not only do we not know whether these cases would be the most complex and needy, but, presumably, some GPs with below-average lists could have no priority cases at all. Strathdee (1992) suggests (on the basis of a 1981 report from the Royal College of General Practitioners) that 55 chronic cases will present during one year. Since there is such a disparity in these figures, we are perhaps best advised to regard Kendrick's empirical work as the best currently available.

Kendrick's 1991 survey of 326 GPs used a definition of long-term mental illness which focused on the group of patients with severe and long-term illness who were in need of long-term intensive supervision. The results showed that the proportion of GPs having more than sixteen cases on their list was only 17 per cent, and only 14 per cent had between eleven and fifteen cases; while 38 per cent had between six and ten cases and 31 per cent had up to five cases. So about 60 per cent have up to ten cases (the average list size was 2,010). In a later study of sixteen practices (Kendrick et al., 1994), the rate of long-term severe illness was found to be three per thousand registered patients. An average list size of 2,300 patients gives a figure of seven cases, which falls within the modal range of his previous work. In addition, 58 per cent of the 253 patients identified in this study had a diagnosis of psychosis, and a higher prevalence of psychotic illness was associated with a higher level of social deprivation.

For the average GP there is a similar problem in respect of the new cases presented during a year. Davies points out that the GP will bring their diagnostic skills to bear on one new schizophrenic case each year. Table 8.2 indicates that the distribution of diagnoses in general practice (level 3) is quite dissimilar to that in secondary care (level 4), reflecting the different levels of the Goldberg/Huxley model. This table also shows that more severe disorder rapidly progresses through the primary care filters.

Table 8.2. Diagnostic conditions at primary and secondary levels of care

Diagnosis	Level 3 %	Level 4 %	Level 5 %
Organic	2	13	15
Schizophrenia	2	20	22
Affective psychosis	3	7	13
Depression	28	27	20
Neurosis	35	12	5
Alcohol/drug	3	7	12
Adjustment disorder, etc.	26	8	4

It comes as no surprise, then, to see the GP's view of who is best placed to care for these patients and who should take the lead in the coordination of their care. Kendrick examined the percentage agreement with statements about the care of people with long-term severe mental illness. Eighty-two per cent agreed with the statement that their care should 'primarily be the responsibility of the psychiatric team'. Half this figure agreed with the statement that the GP should be primarily responsible, with backup from the psychiatric team (41 per cent). A similar pattern emerged in response to the question who should monitor for relapse, with 71 per cent agreeing with this being the responsibility of the psychiatrist and 48 per cent that of the GP. Ninety per cent of the respondents agreed with the idea of shared care.

In respect of their attitudes to these patients, the majority thought that they posed communication problems between the doctor and patient (64 per cent); created a lot of work (68 per cent); caused problems for their families (89 per cent); and only came to attention in a crisis (78 per cent). Almost 40 per cent of them thought that they had a poor prognosis whatever you did (39 per cent), or thought they were better off in hospital (38 per cent). Unsurprisingly, they resisted the role of keyworker, which most (83 per cent) thought should go to the CPN. Social workers were identified as the most appropriate keyworkers by 43 per cent, and only 16 per cent of GPs thought that the patient should rely on the GP as the keyworker.

So, what did they think they should be responsible for? Nearly all (93 per cent) agreed with the idea that the patient's physical problems should be managed by the GP, and almost 80 per cent wanted physical screening done by the GP. Less than half this number (37 per cent) wanted physical screening done by the psychiatrist.

It is clear from various pieces of research that the outcome in both cases of severe long-term disorder and common disorder is better when health and social care are provided in an integrated way (Goldberg and Huxley, 1980; Huxley et al., 1992). To what extent is this a feature of general practice? There are two main sources of data here: Kendrick's survey and a survey by Thomas and Corney (1992) of 261 practices. Although the questions asked were different (about 'attachments' to the practice in Thomas and Corney, and about 'visits' to the practice in Kendrick) the pattern is consistent, in that the CPN was the most commonly attached professional (34 per cent of GPs) and the one who visited most practices (59 per cent). Consultants visited in 37 per cent of practices, social workers in 28 per cent and clinical psychologists in 19 per cent. Social workers were attached to only 6 per cent of practices and counsellors to 17 per cent, although this figure is certainly much higher now.

In 1985, Mitchell reviewed schemes involving psychiatrists in primary care settings and expressed some reservations about extending collaborative arrangements. He commented on the absence of adequate research and evaluation of the various arrangements. Evidence which has been produced since 1985 does not paint a very encouraging picture. For instance, Darling and Tyrer (1990) found that 71 per cent of the contacts between psychiatrists and primary care workers lasted less than five minutes. Anecdotal evidence from many different services suggests that some GPs consult a CPN instead of seeking a psychiatric opinion. The Audit Commission (1994) reports findings (from one district only) which show that social workers' caseloads contained a higher proportion of the severely mentally ill priority group than did CPNs' caseloads. White (1991) reported that, nationally, 25 per cent of CPNs have no schizophrenia sufferers on their caseloads.

The tendency for CPNs to drift away from work with people with severe disorders is marked but not universal. The growth in the use of counsellors and others to provide for people with common disorders is also marked, especially over the past ten years (Waydenfeld and Waydenfeld, 1980; Paykel, 1990). This growth has occurred in the absence of substantial evidence that counselling is effective for all referred groups. Ashurst (quoted in Corney, 1990) randomly assigned patients to counsellors. There was little difference between the counselled and uncounselled groups in terms of relief from symptoms, drug consumption or consultation time with the GP. Brodaty and Andrews (1983), in a study with a small number of subjects, found no differences in symptoms or social outcome between subjects receiving brief psychotherapy, GP counselling and no treatment. Since that time a number of studies have been conducted, which all examine different approaches to the provision of counselling by different professional groups. Corney (1990) has reviewed these and concludes that the evidence for effectiveness is better than it was in the past, but remains mixed (Robson et al., 1984; Teasdale et al., 1984; Johnstone and Shepley, 1986; McLeod, 1988; Holden et al., 1989).

So, in summary, what can be said about the role of the GP in the assessment, treatment and care of mentally ill people? There appears to be an inescapable assessment role, because most people choose this route to present their symptoms. The GP's approach to the treatment of common disorder (if they recognise it) is to prescribe medication and a variety of psychosocial interventions. Research has shown that the prescribing of hypnotics and tranquillisers can be greatly reduced without detriment to the patient (Catalan et al., 1984). The most common forms of psychosocial intervention — the CPN and counsellors — have produced mixed evidence for effectiveness, whereas studies of the less used professionals — especially clinical psychologists and social workers — have shown that they can make a difference (Huxley et al., 1989; Corney, 1990).

At the other end of the spectrum, there is generally a low prevalence of chronic severe illness on the average list, and a low incidence of psychotic illness. Episodes of psychosis tend to be referred rapidly to secondary services, and GPs are not, on the whole, anxious to assume the primary responsibility for their mental health care, and do not wish to be keyworkers. One might argue, and I think I would wish to, that for GPs to treat common disorder, but without medicalising the patient's problems unnecessarily, is appropriate; for them to provide physical health screening is certainly worthwhile; and for them to show a marked reluctance to become involved intensively with a very small number of long-term severely ill patients as keyworker is entirely justified.

The consequences for the purchasing and providing of mental health care which flow from the acceptance of these arguments is beyond the scope of the present chapter, but suggest that some aspects of present government policy are, at best, misconceived. New roles for secondary health care are worthy of further consideration.

What happens when secondary health care is moved into the primary setting?

Given the findings just reviewed, it comes as no surprise to see what happens in practice when secondary care services are offered in a more accessible way to GPs. Figure 8.3 shows the impact of the introduction of a team of accessible mental health professionals in a community

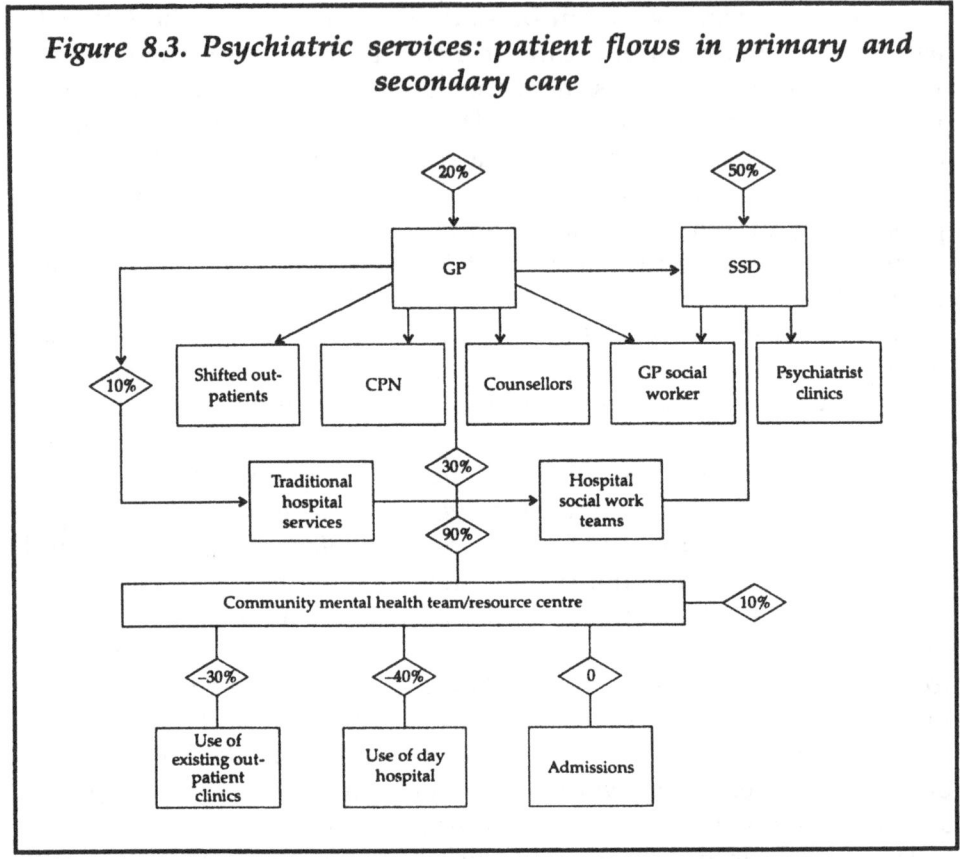

Figure 8.3. Psychiatric services: patient flows in primary and secondary care

setting. The usual referral patterns and use of psychiatric services are affected by the change. The most noticeable alteration, however, is the significant and substantial increase in the numbers of people referred to the community-based psychiatric service who suffer common disorders. The next most evident point is the failure of this approach to affect admissions to hospital.

So, although there is somewhat greater horizontal integration in the team/resource centre, there is little attendant vertical integration. Moreover, there are perverse incentives towards the purchasing of services for common problems, with several potential inefficiencies as a result. Four potential problems could be: the failure to purchase a sufficient number of beds for severely ill people; the purchase of psychosocial interventions which are ineffective or offered to the wrong patients; the absence of incentives to purchase the appropriate combinations of health and social care for long-term groups; and a lack of appropriate mechanisms for purchasing services for conditions of very low prevalence (such as hearing-impaired mentally ill people).

Lessons from the Darlington Project

Given the context outlined earlier, there are a number of areas where the Darlington Project offers lessons of relevance.

Management, administrative arrangements and budgets have to be managed jointly and integrated where possible

At the moment it is not possible to move all mental health funds into a single budget. However, administrative arrangements and management structures are more malleable. Goering and Cochrane (1992) have argued that one of the main critical success factors in initiating changes in mental health service systems is the consolidation of administrative, financial and clinical responsibilities within unified authorities. Achieving joint structures appears to be a worthwhile struggle. Joint managers have a positive effect on the pace of progress of schemes such as the Darlington Project and some mental health schemes (Huxley and Oliver, 1993, 1995).

The importance of targeting

The greater integration of services, especially vertical integration, depends in part upon the specificity with which the target group can be identified. Elsewhere (Huxley, 1991), it has been suggested that, in some mental health programmes in the UK, our current conceptions of a narrowly-defined target group actually lack sufficient specificity. As the Darlington Project confirms, greater specificity contributes to better case-finding and screening performance.

Coordination of care demands clinical case management

Because many of the needs of the long-term care groups with complex problems are social, they will require case management. As I have documented elsewhere (Huxley, 1993), and as the PSSRU work has shown, the case management which is needed is clinical rather than administrative. A long-term relationship with a case manager is a critical component in the survival in a community setting of people with severe mental illness and complex needs.

There are several potential sources of legitimacy for case management

When the object is the improvement of the coordination of care in the mixed economy, then legitimacy for case managers must come from somewhere other than from their employment status in the monopoly or statutory provider. The Darlington Project demonstrates aspects of the other important sources of legitimacy. First, acquiring devolved budgets is an important aspect of flexible community-based care. It is one of the major sources of legitimacy for case managers who, in some other schemes, may not be employed by the major statutory service provider; a budget gives them some purchasing control and financial legitimacy. Second, where integrated services are not feasible or where the law is an obstacle (such as where it mandates the separate provision of health and social care, for instance) then inter-organisational arrangements, such as those involved in joint commissioning, are important sources of legitimacy for case managers. Finally, and somewhat surprisingly, membership of a multidisciplinary team itself constitutes a source of legitimacy. Members of these teams trade their functions in the interests of the needs of different clients. This is usually an informal arrangement, but is mediated in successful teams by powerful aspects of joint working such as trust and loyalty. This type of legitimacy is particularly important in mental health work, and it was noticeable that the case managers were regarded as part of the team in the Darlington Project.

Of course, it may be that in a mixed economy of welfare a single source of legitimacy, such as mandated employment by a monopolistic statutory provider as we had in the UK before the reforms, is insufficient.

More than one source may be required in order to function successfully; exactly how many sources of legitimacy are required for 'success', and of what type and intensity, is a subject for further empirical enquiry.

Conclusions

Challis and his colleagues (1995) have produced a hierarchy of levels at which integration or coordination can take place. In the Darlington scheme there was evidence of collaboration or integration at each of the levels. The matrix, shown in Table 8.3, combines these levels as outlined by Challis et al. (1995), with the concepts of functional integration and collaboration.

Integration is achieved at the agency/management level through mechanisms such as the Joint Boards in Northern Ireland, and through multidisciplinary teams at the professional level. At the agency/ management level in the Darlington scheme, the coordinating group included clinicians; it had to develop an agreed target group and operational policy; and it acted as a forum for the examination of

Table 8.3. Integration-collaboration matrix

	Integrated entities	*Collaborative mechanisms*	*Coordinated functions*	*Examples*
Agency	Northern Ireland Boards	Joint commissioning team	Planning/ spending	Joint finance/ MISG[a]
Professions	Multi-discipline team	Supervisor	Joint management	CPA-CM[b]
Case	Case management	Keyworker	Care coordination	Supervised discharge
Task	Support worker	Combined functions	Support at home	Bathing

a Mental Illness Specific Grant.
b Care Programme Approach – Care Management.

interagency working. At the professional level, the multidisciplinary team included the case managers, and the case reviews contained input from the front-line workers.

At the case level, case management integrates the assessment, care planning, monitoring and direct care functions. In the Darlington scheme the case manager's task was to see that the key case management tasks were undertaken. Screening was undertaken by the case managers so that a targeted service was achieved. At the individual level, support workers integrated the tasks previously discharged by separate workers.

As Moore (1990) has argued, the degree of horizontal integration of services to individuals achieved by case management practice, through coordinating care, needs a degree of vertical integration of client-level work with more strategic concerns at system level in order to be effective.

In conclusion, one might enter a plea that community care should be more like dancing: that is, a vertical expression of a horizontal desire.

References

Audit Commission (1994) *Finding a Place: A Review of Mental Health Services for Adults*, HMSO, London.

Blacker, C.V.R. and Clare, A.W. (1987) Depressive disorder in primary care, *British Journal of Psychiatry*, 150, 737-51.

Bowers, J., Jorm, A.F., Henderson, S. and Harris, P. (1990) General practitioners' detection of depression and dementia in elderly patients, *Medical Journal of Australia*, 153, 4, 192-6.

Bridges, K. and Goldberg, D.P. (1992) Somatisation in primary health care: prevalence and determinants, in B. Cooper and R. Eastwood (eds) *Primary Health Care and Psychiatric Epidemiology*, Routledge, London.

Brodaty, H. and Andrews, G. (1983) Brief psychotherapy in family practice: a controlled prospective intervention trial, *British Journal of Psychiatry*, 143, 11-19.

Catalan, J., Gath, D., Edmonds, G. and Ennis, J. (1984) The effects of non-prescribing of anxiolytics in general practice. I. Controlled evaluation of psychiatric and social outcome, *British Journal of Psychiatry*, 144, 593-602.

Challis, D.J., Darton, R.A., Johnson, L., Stone, M. and Traske, K.J. (1995) *Care Management and Health Care of Older People: The Darlington Community Care Project*, Arena, Aldershot.

Corney, R. (1990) Counselling in general practice – does it work?, *Journal of the Royal Society of Medicine*, 83, 253-7.

Darling, C. and Tyrer, P. (1990) Brief encounters in general practice: liaison in general practice psychiatry clinics, *Psychiatric Bulletin*, 14, 592-4.

Davies, T.M. (1992) Schizophrenia: issues for general practice, in R. Jenkins, V. Field and R. Young (eds) *The Primary Care of Schizophrenia*, HMSO, London.

Giel, R., Koeter, M.W.J. and Ormel, J. (1990) Detection and referral of primary care patients with mental health problems: the second and third filter, in D.P. Goldberg and D. Tantam (eds) *The Public Health Impact of Mental Disorder*, Hogrefe and Huber, Toronto.

Goering, P. and Cochrane, J. (1992) *Critical Success Factors for Mental Health Reform: Lessons for Other Jurisdictions*, Clarke Institute Consulting Group, Toronto.

Goldberg, D. and Huxley, P.J. (1980) *Mental Illness in the Community: The Pathway to Psychiatric Care*, Tavistock, London.

Goldberg, D. and Huxley, P.J. (1992) *Common Mental Disorders: A Biosocial Model*, Routledge, London.

Holden, J.M., Sagovsky, R. and Cox, J.L. (1989) Counselling in a general practice setting: controlled study of health visitor intervention in treatment of postnatal depression, *British Medical Journal*, 298, 223-6.

Huxley, P.J. (1991) Effective case management for mentally ill people: the relevance of recent evidence from the USA for case management services in the United Kingdom, *Social Work and Social Sciences Review*, 2, 3, 192-203.

Huxley, P.J. (1993) Case management and care management in community care, *British Journal of Social Work*, 23, 4, 365-81.

Huxley, P.J. and Oliver, J.P.J. (1993) Mental health policy in practice: lessons from the All Wales Strategy Mental Illness, *International Journal of Social Psychiatry*, 39, 3, 177-89.

Huxley, P.J. and Oliver, J.P.J. (1995) *Powys Community Mental Health Team: Pilot Evaluation*, Report to Powys Social Services Department, Mental Health Social Work Research Unit, University of Manchester, Manchester.

Huxley, P.J., Mohamad, H., Korer, J., Jacob, C., Raval, H. and Anthony, P. (1989) Psychiatric morbidity in social workers' clients: social outcome, *Social Psychiatry and Psychiatric Epidemiology*, 24, 258-65.

Johnstone, A. and Shepley, M. (1986) The outcome of hidden neurotic illness treated in general practice, *Journal of the Royal College of General Practitioners*, 36, 290, 413-15.

Kendrick, T. (1992) The shift to community mental health care: the impact on general practitioners, in R. Jenkins, V. Field and R. Young (eds) *The Primary Care of Schizophrenia*, HMSO, London.

Kendrick, T., Burns, T., Freeling, P. and Sibbald, B. (1994) Provision of care to general practice patients with disabling long-term mental illness: a survey in 16 practices, *British Journal of General Practice*, 44, 384, 301-5.

McLeod, J. (1988) *The Work of Counsellors in General Practice*, Occasional Paper 37, Royal College of General Practitioners, London.

Mari, J. de J., Iacoponi, E., Williams, P., Simoes, O. and Silva, J.B. (1987) Detection of psychiatric morbidity in the primary care setting in Brazil, *Revista de Saude Publica*, 21, 6, 501-7.

Mitchell, A.R.K. (1985) Psychiatrists in primary health care settings, *British Journal of Psychiatry*, 147, 371-9.

Moore, S.T. (1990) A social work practice model of case management: the case management grid, *Social Work*, 35, 5, 444-8.

Paykel, E. (1990) Innovations in mental health care in the primary care system, in I.M. Marks and R.A. Scott (eds) *Mental Health Care Delivery: Innovations, Impediments and Implementation*, Cambridge University Press, Cambridge.

Robson, M.H., France, R. and Bland, M. (1984) Clinical psychologist in primary care: controlled clinical and economic evaluation, *British Medical Journal*, 288, 1805-8.

Stansfeld, S.A., Leek, S.A., Travers, W. and Turner T. (1992) Attitudes to community psychiatry among urban and rural general practitioners, *British Journal of General Practice*, 42, 361, 322-5.

Strathdee, G. (1992) The interface between psychiatry and primary care in the management of schizophrenic patients in the community, in R. Jenkins, V. Field and R. Young (eds) *The Primary Care of Schizophrenia*, HMSO, London.

Teasdale, J.D., Fennell, M.J.V., Hibbert, G.A. and Amies, P.L. (1984) Cognitive therapy for major depressive disorder in primary care, *British Journal of Psychiatry*, 144, 400-406.

Thomas, R.V.R. and Corney, R.H. (1992) A survey of links between mental health professionals and general practice in six district health authorities, *British Journal of General Practice*, 42, 362, 358-61.

Thomas, R.V.R. and Corney, R.H. (1993) Working with community mental health professionals: a survey among general practitioners, *British Journal of General Practice*, 43, 375, 417-21.

Waydenfeld, D. and Waydenfeld, S.W. (1980) Counselling in general practice, *Journal of the Royal College of General Practitioners*, 30, 220, 671-7.

White, E. (1991) *The 3rd Quinquennial National Community Psychiatric Nursing Survey*, Department of Nursing, University of Manchester, Manchester.

9 Cost Opportunities and Constraints in Developing Secondary Health Care in the Community

Ken Wright

The Darlington Project provides us with a topical example of switching secondary care from hospital to the community. Here we have an initiative whose life straddles the great organisational changes which have occurred in health and social care services in this country in the early 1990s. Although many of the project's features are specific to its development, the ways in which it was financed and organised, the details of its continuing evolution and the practicalities of moving from a pilot study to a mainstream service provide excellent examples of the cost opportunities and constraints in developing secondary health care in the community.

Cost opportunities

There are two main types of cost opportunities arising from the development of secondary care in the community. The first of these is concerned generally with the shortening of hospital patients' lengths of stay. It has been known for some time that it is possible to reduce length of hospital stay without detriment to the effectiveness of treatment and with reduced costs of patient care (Drummond, 1980). Indeed, what was once a trickle of opportunities has now become a flood with the development of the strategic shift of secondary care from hospital to the community.

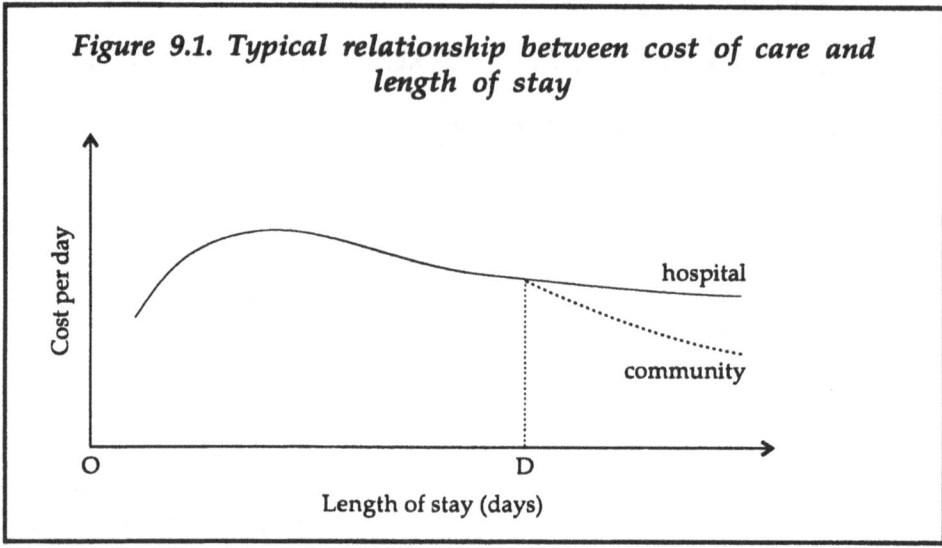

Figure 9.1. Typical relationship between cost of care and length of stay

The typical situation in this example is illustrated in Figure 9.1 where, after some length of stay in hospital for acute care (OD days), it would be possible to care for someone equally effectively but at lower cost in the community. At shorter lengths of stay than OD, it is assumed there is no alternative to acute hospital care because, for example, the patient needs surgery or intensive diagnostic investigation.

The second opportunity arises from the substitution of community-based for continuing care in hospital. This example is illustrated in Figure 9.2, where the costs per day of community-based or hospital care are influenced by the severity of personal care needs. Up to some point, patients with a degree of disability or personal care needs (S in Figure 9.2) can be cared for more cheaply but with at least equal effectiveness in domiciliary care, but after S it is cheaper and at least as effective to care for them in hospital.

Figure 9.2 is intended to simplify the identification of cost opportunities in switching from care in secondary health to community settings. In effect, there are many different forms of continuing care, each with their own cost consequences (Kavanagh et al., 1993), but the example is appropriate to the opportunities and constraints identified in the Darlington Project.

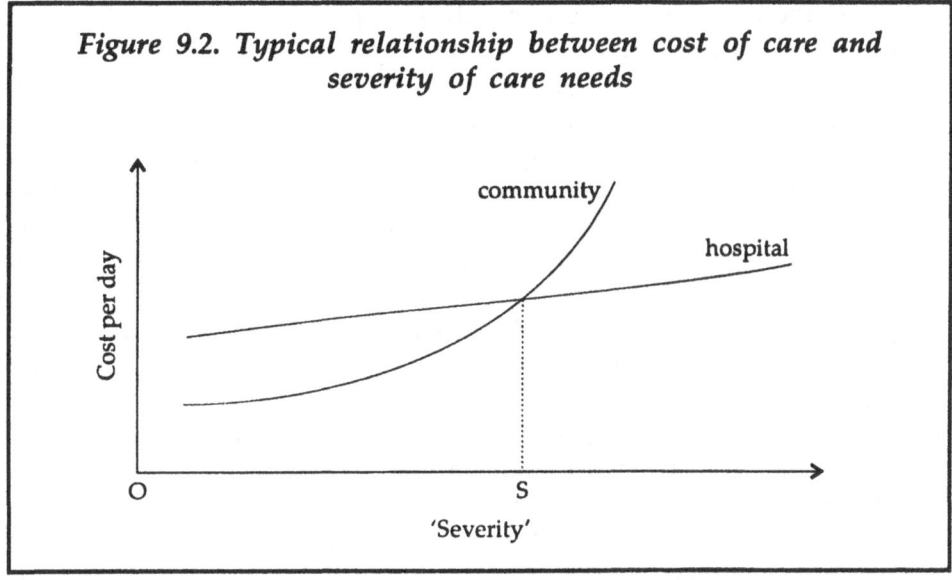

Figure 9.2. Typical relationship between cost of care and severity of care needs

Exploiting the cost opportunities

General issues

There appear to be some general conditions which can make or break initiatives which foster home-based care. First of all, on the economic side it is important to ensure that investment in domiciliary-based care can be paid for by savings in secondary care. This is most likely to occur where the substitution of domiciliary care allows a recognisable and achievable reduction in the need for hospital beds. This does not necessarily mean bed closures; it can also mean avoiding expansion (Gibbins et al., 1982). Resource savings are most likely to occur where a closely-defined population is involved, because it is easier to save on hospital resources when an identifiable set of beds in a ward or a building is involved.

However, it has to be recognised that, at times, it will be necessary to invest in the domiciliary services before the hospital facilities are closed down. Additionally, where domiciliary care substitutes for new-build or other capital expenditure in hospitals, it must be possible to set off increased revenue expenditure against savings in the capital budget. Sometimes this is easily done in the early years of a scheme, but it is easy to lose sight of this two or three years later, when attention is focused on incremental increases in the revenue budget and the reductions in the proposed capital budget have been forgotten. A typical scenario is that intensive domiciliary care is evaluated in the planning cycle against the expansion of hospital care. The domiciliary care expansion falls mainly on the revenue budget, whereas the budgetary implications of avoiding the extension of hospital buildings fall on both revenue and capital budgets. A decision is taken to pursue the intensive domiciliary care option, but as it expands over a few years it becomes a victim of its own success. Its demand for increased revenue spending is compared with the previous years' budgets, while the savings which accrued on the capital budget (capital and revenue budgets are developed separately) are forgotten.

Increased revenue expenditure can also result from the example of reducing lengths of inpatient stays, when the space made available is not left idle but is used by the admission of new patients. If the cost per patient day follows the relationship illustrated in Figure 9.1, the effect of reducing lengths of stay is to replace the cheaper days towards the end of the stay with the more expensive early days, when diagnostic investigations and treatments are more intensive. Although it may well be an efficient and effective way of reducing waiting lists or times, reducing lengths of stay can increase total hospital expenditure. Thus, what is perceived by providers as increased efficiency may be perceived by purchasers as a way of rapidly exhausting their budgets.

Second, one needs a clear statement of responsibilities for the provision of domiciliary care, because it will involve a number of duties which can be equally effectively carried out by personnel from several agencies. A number of intensive domiciliary care schemes have been run by the NHS (Knowelden et al., 1991), local authorities (Latto, 1982) and the independent sector (Gibbs and Wright, 1993). The key working principles appear to be flexibility in being able to carry out a wide range of personal and general caring duties, as well as in covering different times of the day and days of the week. The awkward factor is often whether or not the service user is compelled to pay a service charge.

Third, users and carers need to know where to go when they need help. It follows from this that the development of good domiciliary care requires careful care planning, in terms of assessment of the needs of both users and of carers, the design of effective packages of care and the monitoring of progress, with easy access by users and carers in times of emergency: in other words, the effective implementation of the core tasks of care management (Challis et al., 1995).

Fourth, it is necessary to obtain the cooperation of all the agencies likely to be involved, including primary, secondary and community health services, social services, housing services and the Benefits Agency. Although care managers might well be aware of the need to provide multi-agency packages of care, it is highly unlikely that they will have direct purchasing power to buy in services across such a diverse set of agencies and, therefore, they will be reliant on good interagency planning, coordination and goodwill among purchasers and providers in these different organisations.

Lessons from the Darlington Project

It is interesting to see how the Darlington scheme tackled these issues. First, it was directed towards a specific group of people — physically frail but mentally alert elderly people — who would have used specific facilities, in this case continuing care hospital beds. It is relatively easy, therefore, to identify the facilities that would be freed by caring for this group of people. If the scheme had been directed at people who used a wide range of medical or surgical inpatient facilities spread across several wards or hospitals, it would have been difficult to identify the resources freed and to calculate the marginal cost savings (Knowelden et al., 1991).

Second, the development of the hybrid home care worker provides an excellent example of dealing with the skill mix issue in domiciliary care. As explained in the account of the project (Challis et al., 1995, p.25), the home care assistant's role covered not only home help and home nursing auxiliary tasks, but also those carried out by physiotherapy and occupational therapy helpers. The organisational location of these workers, either in the NHS or in a local authority, is important because of the co-payment issue in local authority services. Generally, one would expect that service users would prefer provision by the health service, because that is free, to a local authority service for which they may be asked to pay. The home care assistants who were still in post at the end of the pilot project signed health service employment contracts, and thereby ensured that service users did not have to make a direct contribution to the costs of the service.

The key role of the core tasks of care management played an important part of the success of the Darlington Project. The care managers clearly faced considerable pressures in meeting the conflicts of interest which arise in intensive domiciliary care, whether it be between the service providers and users, between the frail elderly person and carer, or between service providers from different agencies (Challis et al., 1995, p.98). The determination of a manageable caseload and a supervisory and support network appeared to be crucial factors in assisting care managers to cope with these pressures. This aspect of the project provides very useful insights into the process of establishing and maintaining effective care management on a day-to-day basis.

Closely related to this is the experience of multi-agency working in the project. To some extent interagency cooperation was facilitated by the policy context. The project was part of the government's Care in the Community Initiative and, therefore, had a high national profile and an accompanying evaluation. Nevertheless, local circumstances and staff contributed to the successful implementation. In addition to the resources committed by the health and local authorities in the area, the local housing agencies also played their parts in pledging their support to the venture, although the anticipated housing facilities were not, in fact, made available to the project.

One wonders in the end, though, whether any of this would have worked if the Care in the Community Initiative had not provided the flexible finance to give the project its necessary pump-priming. In today's circumstances, what pot of money would play this role? Generally, it is more likely that such finance would be available if the cost savings accrued to the agency which was financing the new scheme. Before 1990, NHS provision would have met this condition, but after 1990 it is less certain. Much would depend on the attitude of health service purchasers and GP fundholders, and how they would handle transferring contracts from hospital to community health trusts.

Constraints on developing secondary care in the community

The interesting feature of the Darlington Project is that its development covered the period since 1985, and therefore the transition to the reorganisation of health and social care in the early 1990s. How well were the general problems and constraints facing the delivery of health and social care being tackled? The last two chapters of the book are very revealing in this respect, in their coverage of issues such as continued financial support, flexible working arrangements, charging for social care services, continued service coordination and the implementation of the purchaser/provider split. It is very striking to read how the problems of converting the project from a pilot study to a mainstream service highlighted again the criticisms made by the Audit Commission (1986) about the disjointed financial and administrative arrangements which have constrained the development of community care.

A main concern of the Audit Commission and the subsequent report by Sir Roy Griffiths (1988) and the White Paper (Cm 849, 1989) on community care was the way in which the social security budget had been used to finance an enormous increase in private residential or nursing home care for elderly people (Darton and Wright, 1993). This was addressed in the subsequent legislation, and has been put into practice by giving local authorities the responsibility for funding residential and nursing home care for those people who cannot meet the fees from their own resources. However, many of the other issues and problems highlighted still exist. Ring-fencing of community care budgets (apart from the monies transferred from the social security budget) was not implemented, nor was the idea of a specific grant-inaid to local authorities for community care, nor the establishment of single-agency organisation. Consequently, the concern that the funding of community care was bound up with the whole problem of local government finance, with council tax-capping, and with the appropriateness and adequacy of the Standard Spending Assessments for the basis of the general grant still remains, as we have seen recently in financing local education and social services. Moreover, the worries that the Audit Commission expressed over the fragmentation of services have been exacerbated, not so much by the community care aspects of the recent reorganisation of the NHS and community care, as by the creation of NHS trusts, including the separation of community from hospital trusts, and the development of the purchaser/provider split, or the purchaser/ purchaser split following the development of GP fundholders as competitive purchasers of services with district health services. The operation of these constraints is well illustrated in the continued development of the Darlington Project.

Although both health services and social services appeared keen to develop a joint-agency service, joint funding was difficult and the health authority became the single funding agency at the end of the project. However, for general dissemination of such an initiative, it has to be noted that the funding decision was based on savings accruing from the reduced use of NHS continuing care beds, and that attempts to widen the base to social services were not successful. Moreover, in these days of separate NHS provision through hospital or community trusts, and split purchasing responsibilities between health authorities, GP fundholders and social services, even single-agency health service funding could pose problems.

The use of the single NHS-based agency model for the continued provision of the project is interesting because it tackled problems which either a multi-level agency or a local authority single agency might have had difficulty in solving. At the simplest level, it meant that users were not charged for the service, as they would have been with local authority funding. Second, the home care assistants carried out some duties which could easily have been performed by home helps, but also had training to support the therapy professions. This means that the services which complemented the work of the home care assistants were NHS rather than social services-based, and in terms of the pur-chaser/provider split it was sensible to make it a health rather than a social services-provided service. Moreover, as Challis et al. report, 'In these more contentious areas developments may perhaps occur more readily where an agency can singlehandedly act on behalf of both, rather than where there is a continuing dual involvement' (1995, p.292).

Despite the Audit Commission's recommendation, it is unlikely that single-agency working will ever operate in the care of elderly people. There are too many organisations involved (for example, the NHS, local authority social services, housing associations and the Benefits Agency) to make this realistic. There are, however, ways in which cross-agency working might be helped; for example, by using programme budgeting techniques (Jones and Wright, 1995), and by multiprofessional community teams, joint planning and joint commissioning between health and local authorities (Department of Health, 1993). Imaginative workforce policies also help to overcome some of the barriers which have sprung up around the rather artificial division of health from social care.

It was gratifying to read that some of the flexibility of the working arrangements in Darlington were preserved through the retention of the general purpose home care assistants. This was achieved despite some consideration being given to altering the skill mix specification for home care. Fortunately, attempts to 'task' the work of the assistants were unsuccessful and the general principle of an all-purpose, main or sole contact generally prevailed. In these days of local pay determination, especially for health care assistants, the specification of skill mix by task analysis and the focus on labour costs alone, rather than labour productivity (that is, cost and outcome), might well make it difficult to replicate this model of working. Measuring the efficiency and effectiveness of the home care assistants depends on someone being able to assess the quality and outcome of their work with individual clients. The coordination of service provision and the appropriate assessments of client and carer needs became difficult, and this illustrates the general point raised by such schemes, that they need someone to carry out the core tasks of care management in order to ensure that an appropriate package of care is delivered, and changes in client and carer quality of life are monitored.

Conclusion

Whenever organisations are divided or departmentalised, whenever responsibilities for a policy are shared between agencies, whenever financial responsibility covers different organisations, some of whom work to strict budgeting cash limits and others do not, and whenever some people pay for some services that are provided free of charge by other agencies, there are opportunities for innovative collaborative behaviour as well as for the cost-shunting and buck-passing that we have come to recognise in the provision of health and social care for elderly people.

The financial and organisational basis of community care is unlikely to change in the foreseeable future. We have, therefore, to make the best of it. The Darlington Project highlights a set of characteristics which enable one to make progress. These characteristics appear to be:

- a closely defined target group of people who will be eligible for the service, which has kept it out of the more general disputes over continuing care of elderly people in hospital or at home;
- a clear financial focus: a service which allows hospital beds to be used more efficiently;
- clearly-defined organisational arrangements;
- a home care worker who can provide for a large variety of users' needs;
- a clear commitment to keeping out of the semantic squabbles over the definition of health and social care; and
- a set of managers and clinicians keen and able to develop innovatory ways of working together.

A whole range of reactions to the financial and administrative arrangements for community care is possible. Some people may become resigned to the difficulties and constraints in the system and lose their enthusiasm to battle through the maze of financial regulations and organisational and professional divisions. Others will regard the system as a challenge to their inventiveness. The comforting aspect of the Darlington Project is that it shows how creative and innovative opportunism can overcome the potential obstacles of interagency collaboration in the care of very frail elderly people. One of the greatest challenges posed by the development of secondary care in the community is how to convert this type of innovatory scheme into regular service provision. The Care in the Community Initiative provided the necessary pump-priming finance to encourage such schemes. Health and social services purchasers may take a lead from such an example, and set aside a form of joint health and social services funding, which will not only encourage innovatory schemes but also ensure that those developments which have proved their cost-effectiveness can be absorbed into mainstream services.

References

Audit Commission (1986) *Making a Reality of Community Care*, HMSO, London.

Challis, D.J., Darton, R.A., Johnson, L., Stone, M. and Traske, K.J. (1995) *Care Management and Health Care of Older People: The Darlington Community Care Project*, Arena, Aldershot.

Cm 849 (1989) *Caring for People: Community Care in the Next Decade and Beyond*, HMSO, London.

Darton, R.A. and Wright, K.G. (1993) Changes in the provision of long-stay care, 1970-1990, *Health and Social Care in the Community*, 1, 1, 11-25.

Department of Health (1993) *Implementing Community Care: Joint Commissioning for Community Care: "A Slice Through Time"*, Department of Health, London.

Drummond, M.F. (1980) *Principles of Economic Appraisal in Health Care*, Oxford University Press, Oxford.

Gibbins, F.J., Lee, M., Davison, P.R., O'Sullivan, P., Hutchinson, M., Murphy, D.R. and Ugwu, C.N. (1982) Augmented home nursing as an alternative to hospital care for chronic elderly invalids, *British Medical Journal*, 284, 330-33.

Gibbs, I. and Wright, K.G. (1993) *Anchor Care Team: An Appraisal*, Anchor Housing Trust, Oxford.

Griffiths, R. (1988) *Community Care: Agenda for Action*, A Report to the Secretary of State for Social Services, HMSO, London.

Jones, C. and Wright, K.G. (1995) *Programme Budgeting Revisited: Special Reference to People with Learning Disabilities*, Discussion Paper 127, Centre for Health Economics, University of York, York.

Kavanagh, S., Schneider, J., Knapp, M.R.J., Beecham, J.K. and Netten, A.P. (1993) Elderly people with cognitive impairment: costing possible changes in the balance of care, *Health and Social Care in the Community*, 1, 2, 69-80.

Knowelden, J., Westlake, L., Wright, K.G. and Clarke, S.J. (1991) Peterborough Hospital-at-Home, *Journal of Public Health Medicine*, 13, 182-8.

Latto, S. (1982) *The Coventry Home Help Project*, Coventry Social Services Department, Coventry.

10 Linking Community Care and Health Care: A New Role for Secondary Health Care Services

David Challis, Robin Darton and Karen Stewart

The provision of effective long-term care at home for frail older people requires planned and coordinated inputs from health and social care agencies. This is evident from a range of research studies (see, for example, Challis et al., 1995) which indicate the interplay between social care needs and clinical phenomena, and which have been reinforced by policy guidance. For example, although the level of functional impairment is an important influence upon the probability of placement in residential settings, so too is the presence of certain diagnoses (Tsuji et al., 1995; Darton et al., 1997). Rockwood et al. (1996) found that entry to a long-term care facility was associated not only with social factors and functional difficulties, such as female gender, being unmarried, the absence of a caregiver, the presence of cognitive impairment and functional impairment, but also with clinical diagnoses, such as diabetes mellitus, stroke and Parkinson's disease. They concluded that frailty is multidimensional and not simply a synonym for dependence in activities of daily living. Furthermore, the importance of the psychosocial needs of older people and their carers as determinants of placement has been identified in several studies (Jorm et al., 1993; Tsuji et al., 1995). For some individuals, particularly those with complex needs, a primary health care-led NHS may be insufficient, lacking both the range and depth of response necessary. The key question, therefore, is how to combine what kinds of inputs, whether primary or secondary, health or social, for which individuals, in what ways.

The chapters in this book address important aspects of this key question. There is broad agreement on the interdependence of health and social care, and a recognition that, at least for some individuals, a more complex response, traditionally associated with secondary care, may be essential for the effective maintenance of older people in the community. Some chapters specifically describe the nature of service level activities which attempt to transcend these divisions, linking health and social care or secondary care with social care. These relate to aspects of need with a relatively low prevalence among the patients on the list of any one general practitioner, but whose level of need is likely to be high in terms of the consumption of resources or the generation of public concern, and for whom primary care may not be the most appropriate locus for their support.

Changes in both the health care system and within social care services necessitate a re-evaluation of service configurations. In health care, one factor propelling secondary health care towards a new role is the reduction in NHS continuing care provision, and the consequent need to maintain in the community some individuals who would previously have received this form of care. Another factor is the reduction in the average hospital length of stay, with the consequence that people may be discharged with continuing treatment and rehabilitation requirements which would previously have been met by hospital care. Instead, they may be discharged to social and community health care services whose capacity and resources have lagged behind the current demands placed upon them.

In the field of social care, the reconsideration of the nature of care management is an important factor. Following the 1990 NHS and Community Care Act, care management was implemented in a relatively broad and generic fashion, but there has been a growing tendency to consider more differentiated forms which reflect the needs of older people in different circumstances (Department of Health, 1994a). As care management becomes more differentiated, the more intensive forms of care management for people with severe and complex needs (Challis, 1994) need to make appropriate linkages with health care provision, which will often be secondary health care services. Hence, there is a clear link between the development of secondary health care in the community and intensive care management.

In the rest of this chapter, we examine the potential relationship between secondary health care and care management in terms of a number of key themes which have been raised consistently in the previous chapters, all of which are critical for the development of community care into the 21st century. These are: assessment, rehabilitation, care management, and the integration of health and social care.

Assessment

Assessment was identified as one of the cornerstones of community care in the 1989 White Paper *Caring for People* (Cm 849, 1989), and was made a prerequisite prior to publicly-funded placement in care homes. Similarly, in Australia, the concern for more appropriate targeting of places in nursing homes is reflected in the focus upon the improvement of assessment processes at the point of entry to long-term care. However, the content of assessment processes is immensely variable. In Australia, Geriatric Assessment Teams, which are often full multidisciplinary groupings, are responsible for the pre-placement assessment, whereas no such formal arrangement for a joint health and social care assessment is prescribed in the UK community care reforms, although recent guidance requires authorities to consider this further (Department of Health, 1997).

Comprehensive Geriatric Assessment (CGA) has been described as including functional status, mental and physical health, identification of disease and dysfunction, specification of appropriate treatments and intervention, assessment of the need for support services, evaluation of the effects of intervention and monitoring of the effects upon quality of life (Rubenstein et al., 1988). This strategy is by no means new and much is founded upon the work of Marjory Warren. Among the factors seen as critical for success were: a positive approach; individual patient assessment; patient involvement; team working; and maximising independence through optimising the patient's environment (Warren, 1946). The specialty of geriatric medicine formally recognised the interdependence of physical, psychological and social problems, requiring comprehensive assessment (Isaacs, 1981). The effectiveness of the approach can be seen in consequent improvements in the outcome of health care (Stuck et al., 1993). Studies have indicated that CGA uncovers a range of unidentified health needs (Rubenstein et al., 1994), such as cognitive impairment, depression and incontinence, and can reduce carer stress (Silverman et al., 1995).

This strategy of comprehensive assessment needs to be employed at major transition points in the care of older people, such as the decision whether or not to enter residential or nursing home care. One of the first studies to examine this was that of Brocklehurst and colleagues (1978), who found that, of 100 referrals to local authority residential homes, seventeen did not require this level of care when fully assessed and investigated. Similar conclusions may be drawn from other, more recent work. In a randomised trial of specialist assessment compared with the usual process in the United States, Applegate et al. (1990) found that geriatric assessment could improve function, decrease risk of nursing home placement and reduce mortality. In a trial of in-home assessment for older people living in the community in Switzerland, Stuck et al. (1995) found that it reduced the development of disability and reduced permanent nursing home stays. In the UK, Peet et al. (1994) assessed 117 applicants for residential care, of whom 63 were medically examined and offered intervention if deemed appropriate. Intervention appeared to redirect some applicants to more appropriate forms of care, and resulted in improved levels of psychological well-being. Secondly, Sharma et al. (1994) supplemented the usual assessment of applicants for residential accommodation with a formal multidisciplinary clinical assessment at a rehabilitation centre. Of 199 cases, clinical assessment detected apparently unknown medical problems in 158 elderly people, most of which were amenable to treatment. Of the 173 cases recommended for residential care on the basis of social work assessment alone, 49 were judged to be better placed elsewhere following clinical assessment. The authors suggest that the findings make a clear case for a programme of formal clinical assessment prior to placement. Thirdly, Peet et al. (1996) assessed the management of urinary incontinence among older people in residential and nursing homes. They found a high prevalence of severe and uncontrolled symptoms of urinary incontinence, combined with a lack of support provided to the homes for the management of such residents, which indicated a need for a greater specialist service input for more effective care.

The new community care legislation and the expectation of the development of intensive packages of care have increased the importance of detailed assessment of older people for the receipt of community care (Audit Commission, 1997). The chapter in this book by Iain Carpenter provides an example of a development towards more systematic home care assessment systems. This is of crucial importance, since many of the critical indicators of need are often missed by general practitioners, as the chapter by Huxley indicates. The classic study by Williamson and colleagues (1964) indicated levels of morbidity in older people which were unknown to general practitioners. In particular, dementia is frequently not recognised in primary care (Ineichen, 1994). More recent work has noted that depressive disorders, which are present in significant numbers of older people receiving home care (Banerjee and Macdonald, 1996), are frequently not recognised by home care staff (Dalton and Busch, 1995). This is particularly significant in the light of evidence that specialist secondary services appear to be able to offer a more effective response to older people with depression (Banerjee et al., 1996).

There is clear evidence that frail older people have unmet care needs, which are often undiagnosed by primary health and social care workers. Furthermore, it is clear that systematic evaluation of frail older people by secondary health care services can yield significant gains, in terms of functioning, the prevention of inappropriate placement and more effective management of care. Under the current community care arrangements, a large number of admissions to residential and nursing homes are made directly from hospital settings. This could provide a means for undertaking more systematic, opportunistic clinical evaluation of patients prior to placement by specialist secondary services. The studies reviewed above suggest the possibility of real gain from this process, particularly when, as in opportunistic evaluation (Bowns et al., 1991), the assessment would be undertaken at marginal rather than average cost.

Care management

Much of the concern about the development of care management following the implementation of the 1990 Act in the UK relates to the emergence of a relatively generic and non-specific approach, which was not clearly targeted (Department of Health, 1994a). Bob Welch addresses this issue in the second chapter of this book. Debates have taken place as to whether care management is described as a role undertaken by specific staff, or as a process through which most service users should pass as a means of accessing the forms of care they require. In order to disentangle these debates it is necessary to differentiate both the form of care management and the roles of staff. The sixth annual report of the Chief Inspector of the Social Services Inspectorate makes the need for differentiation explicit (SSI, 1997). It suggested that part of the explanation for the problems encountered with the volume and flow of work faced by social services may be partly attributable to a failure to differentiate between levels of intervention. Three types or styles of care management were specified as appropriate for different levels of response, the range of responses being necessary for an integrated and comprehensive approach to the provision of care:

- the administrative type, undertaken by reception and/or customer service staff, provides information and advice;
- the coordinating type that deals with a large volume of referrals needing either a single service or a range of fairly straightforward services which should be properly planned and administered; and
- the intensive type where there is a designated care manager who combines the planning and coordination with a therapeutic, supportive role for a much smaller number of users who have complex and frequently changing needs.
(SSI, 1997, para 3.4.)

The lack of differentiation and the emergence of more generic models was judged to result from a failure to discriminate between the coordinating and intensive forms of care management. The Social Services Inspectorate states that 'The crucial objectives are to ensure that long term care management is devoted to those people who need it and that decisions about the skills of staff to be deployed and about monitoring and reviewing arrangements reflect this' (SSI, 1997, para 3.5). Of course, these debates are not new. What is new is more explicit guidance about how authorities need to shape their response in a differentiated fashion. In the Department of Health monitoring studies of the early implementation of assessment and care management, three distinct approaches were evident: the designated care manager; care management as a role within an existing job; and a dual role with staff designated to work part time as designated care manager and part time as social worker

(Department of Health, 1993, 1994a). In some work undertaken for the Scottish Office, Buglass (1993) cites three similar models: care management as a separate job; care management as a role within an existing job and within an existing agency; and care management as a role within a joint health and social care structure. The more that care management is viewed as a role within an existing job or as a description of the organisational process, the greater the probability of a more generic, and undifferentiated style of service.

The distinction between the role of key worker and the role of care manager may be helpful in differentiating between the coordinating and the intensive care management roles. Several factors have been identified which discriminate between these two activities (Challis et al., 1995). These include the intensity of involvement, the breadth of services spanned and the duration of involvement (Applebaum and Austin, 1990). Care management aims to coordinate multiple services and providers, usually on a long-term basis, whereas a keyworker would have a more short-term, less intensive and narrower range of responsibilities, reflected by factors such as more frequent case turnover. Øvretveit (1993) distinguishes key workers from care managers by reference to the key workers' narrower range of services spanned, usually restricted to the services for which they are directly responsible.

A review of care management in a Scottish local authority noted how authorities have 'taken various steps to define, develop and implement their own versions of [assessment and care management], but what is striking about this, is the absence of any general consensus as to one clear model with which to best deliver the objectives of Community Care' (Scottish Borders Council Social Work Department, 1997, p.3). Department of Health guidance suggests that more than one model is required within any one agency (Department of Health, 1994a). The problems identified in the Scottish report included: a need to focus care management effort on the most appropriate cases; a lack of care management coordination across agencies; a lack of review; and an administrative, rather than a professional form of care management. There would probably be widespread agreement with the findings of this review. The Scottish report identified ten aspects of change, including five which were concerned with ways in which there could be closer integration of other agencies, particularly health, into the care management process; one which was designed to achieve a closer shared vision and interagency consensus; and one which was designed to focus care management upon a more narrowly defined target population. Developing closer links between care management and secondary health care would offer a means of achieving some of these objectives, particularly the development of intensive care management for a narrowly defined target population. This may be contrasted with the pressure to move towards a primary care driven health service (Department of Health and the Welsh Office, 1989). Linking care managers with primary health care does appear to improve access and speed of referral (Russell Hodgson, 1997). However, effective targeting, a differentiated response and access to specialist assessment skills are less readily achieved. The observations in the 1997 Social Services Inspectorate report, the conclusions of a Scottish local authority and the findings of a study of care management in primary care suggest that many of the gains for those people requiring intensive responses may be more readily achieved by undertaking assessment and care management in conjunction with secondary care services, following an initial screening process. The Darlington study, discussed earlier in this book, was such an attempt. To pursue the Social Services Inspectorate's models of care management further: the administrative type represents a need to enhance and improve information, advice and screening systems; the coordinating model can be seen as a primary level response by social care; while the provision of intensive care management can be seen as a secondary level response. Employing the administrative structures, linkages and types of care management specified by the Social Services Inspectorate could do much to tackle the difficulties currently faced by agencies in implementing care management.

Rehabilitation

One feature of current developments in health and social care has been the growing differentiation between long-term care and support provided by social care and acute health care provided by the NHS. One activity with the potential of bridging the two, rehabilitation, is a source of increasing concern, since both its scale and location may be inappropriate for its potential to be fully realised (House of Commons Health Committee, 1995; SSI, 1995). Mulley (1994) suggests that rehabilitation is moving from an earlier focus on younger people, towards the achievement of independence and wellbeing of older people. However, there would appear to be enormous variations in the scale and type of rehabilitation services, which militate against the emergence of a coherent service model (Beardshaw, 1988). Rehabilitation is predominantly focused upon the restoration of function (Beardshaw, 1988; Waters, 1996; Waters and Luker, 1996). Inevitably, much rehabilitative activity has been concentrated on the acute phase of illness and disability, and within a hospital setting (Waters, 1987; Gibbon and Thompson, 1992; Walker, 1995). Nolan (1997) argues that rehabilitation is constrained by the functional model of health prevalent within medicine, which can lead to incomplete care for both older people and their carers. In contrast, however, Wright (1983) notes that achieving greater independence involves improvement in physical functioning, changes in the elderly person's environment and changes in the attitudes of the elderly person and their relations, and, in their chapter in this book, MacMahon and his colleagues emphasise the value of assessment and rehabilitation in maintaining older people in their own homes.

As hospital lengths of stay for older patients are reduced, rehabilitation, linked to community services and discharge programmes, is likely to be increasingly important if services are not to be inappropriately provided to maintain individuals post discharge. Rehabilitation resources are likely to be increasingly required in nursing, residential and other long-term care settings (Department of Health, 1995a; Hastings, 1997). The quality of hospital discharge is an area of increasing importance for effective care (Fairhurst et al., 1996), evident in the detailed guidance on hospital discharge arrangements provided in the Hospital Discharge Workbook (Department of Health, 1994b). A reduction in the length of stay has led to rehabilitation programmes being developed in the United States, based upon the UK model of the day hospital (Evans et al., 1995). Rehabilitation services may be linked to hospital at home provision with some benefit in reduction of length of stay (Donald et al., 1995). Evidence suggests that long-term patients provided with appropriate occupational therapy are able to mobilise latent resources of cognitive and psycho-social performance (Bach et al., 1995). Elderly people in residential care settings improved in both balance and functional performance following individualised physical therapy training programmes (Harada et al., 1995). Studies of patients with stroke suggest the importance of continuing rehabilitation following discharge (Garraway et al., 1980; Young and Forster, 1992; Young, 1994; Gladman et al., 1995). Similar judgements can be made about orthopaedic services, where there is evidence that patients with fractured neck of femur may be cared for in community settings with associated rehabilitation at lower costs than for hospital care (Hollingworth et al., 1993; Farnworth et al., 1994).

Rehabilitation, therefore, has increasingly to be seen as part of the process of managing hospital discharge for frail older people. There is evidence that more focused, specialist services are most effective in promoting discharge. A trial of an augmented home help service to assist in the discharge from acute hospital beds of older patients who experienced social problems proved largely unsuccessful, with no evidence of either speedier discharge or improvements in wellbeing (Victor and Vetter, 1988). This was attributed to the relatively small additional elements of service being insufficient for the wide range of needs identified. More successful discharge programmes have been more tightly focused, specialised and linked to secondary health care services. Townsend et al. (1988) found that a service with care assistants providing help for up to twelve hours per week for a two week period after discharge, and undertaking a range of personal, domestic and therapeutic tasks, was markedly more effective than standard aftercare. The number of days spent in hospital by those receiving the service was significantly reduced compared with a control population. Martin et al. (1994) evaluated a high support hospital discharge scheme for older people. Those receiving input from the home treatment team had fewer readmissions, spent fewer days in hospital and remained at home longer than a control population. The linking of rehabilitation and hospital discharge suggests further opportunities for the developing relationship between secondary health care and community-based care. One feature of more differentiated care management could be the development of separate systems for long-term care management and hospital discharge. This is in contrast to the merging of the two, as has tended to occur, with relatively more effort being placed on the hospital discharge process than the provision of long-term care at home (Department of Health, 1994a).

Health and social care

The boundary between health and social care has never been easy to identify or define precisely. Drawing upon a study undertaken by the National Association of Health Authorities and Trusts, the 1991 guidance on care management listed 24 groups of tasks relevant to the care of older people which could be used to clarify the respective responsibilities of health and social care, and indicate where joint provision could be developed. Of these tasks, six were recorded as health care tasks and seven as social care tasks, while the remaining eleven were definable as the province of either health or social care (SSI/SWSG, 1991). If the distinction between health and social care is more a result of administrative history than of rational definition, the attempt to create boundaries by identifying distinct and sectorally unique tasks is likely to be extremely difficult, and ultimately fruitless.

An alternative strategy to the precise distinction of roles and tasks is to consider mechanisms of integration. This requires clarification of the nature of processes of integration. There are distinctly different forms of linking or integrating agencies. An insight may be gained by using an analogy from the literature of economics. It is possible to distinguish two different forms of integration, horizontal integration and vertical integration. Horizontal integration may be defined as the integration of activities which occur at the same level in the production process. It consists of integration by the control, or ownership, of processes not sequentially linked but complementary to one another. For example, one retail organisation may acquire another or, in health care terms, an acute trust may undertake to provide an additional acute care specialty, alongside those currently provided. By contrast, vertical integration may be defined as the integration of different stages or processes associated with the same final product. For example, an automobile manufacturer may acquire steel production or retail facilities, and either would constitute greater vertical integration. In health care terms, an acute trust may integrate with a community trust to provide greater continuity of health care, from in-patient care through early discharge programmes to care at home. Alternatively, though much less plausible, an acute care trust may acquire control of fundholding GPs so as to integrate vertically their source of supply of patients with hospital care provision. Using these two concepts it is helpful to look again at the mechanisms by which government has attempted to bring together health and social care.

The history of attempts to link health and social care could be seen as attempts to achieve greater horizontal integration, that is, to link together two organisations operating at the same stage in the production process of care for older people. The pursuit of vertical integration is less evident. The long history of joint planning, emphasising exhortation (Webb and Wistow, 1986), can be seen as part of the attempt to achieve horizontal integration. Similarly, the requirement upon agencies to develop hospital discharge arrangements just prior to the full implementation of the 1990 NHS and Community Care Act (Department of Health, 1992) can be characterised as linking processes perceived as parallel rather than as sequential. The guidance for the production of community care plans (Department of Health, 1995b) is a more recent example which emphasises horizontal more than vertical integration.

Nonetheless, there is evidence in central guidance of the importance of vertical integration:

> In some instances, intensive care at home may be more appropriate than a residential or nursing home admission. Health authorities/ boards and social services/social work authorities may wish to co-operate in establishing multi-disciplinary teams for geriatric and psycho-geriatric care, similar to those which already exist in the fields of mental health and mental handicap, to develop innovative forms of intensive domiciliary care. Where this involves care that was previously provided in a hospital setting, the responsibilities of consultant teams and general practitioners will need to be re-negotiated. Similar negotiations will be required where hospital-based practitioners become involved in maintaining patients in the community. (SSI/SSWG, 1991, para. 4.43.)

There are some examples of approaches to integration between health and social care which follow more closely the emphasis on vertical integration. The Darlington Project, described in Chapter 4, was an attempt to provide more integrated health and social care by linking care managers with budgetary responsibility and control of the time of multipurpose home care assistants with a geriatric multidisciplinary team (Challis et al., 1995). Similarly, the Lewisham Intensive Case Management Scheme (Challis et al., 1997) provided a link between care managers and a community mental health team for the elderly, providing diagnosis, assessment and continuing care at home. In an earlier chapter, MacMahon and his colleagues have described the CARTs Project, which linked community-based assessment with the provision of rehabilitation. Another example of vertical integration of rehabilitation and home care can be seen in the Gloucester Hospital-at-Home rehabilitation service, which was linked to in-patient orthopaedic care (Donald et al., 1995). There have also been a number of studies which have examined the gain of specialist assessment at the point of transition in an elderly person's life between home care and residential or nursing home care (Brocklehurst et al., 1978; Peet et al., 1994; Sharma et al., 1994). On a broader scale, the arrangements in Northern Ireland provide an example of an integrated service provider, where a single community trust provides community health and social care. This could be seen as combining aspects of horizontal integration, through the provision of a wide range of care, from child care to social care of older people, with vertical integration through a single funder and integrated provider of health and social care, offering diagnosis, assessment, treatment and community care services.

A trend towards the emphasis on vertical integration as a means of making sense of the complex relationship between health and social care may be identified elsewhere. In Sweden the relationship between health and social care was traditionally seen as one of unclear responsibilities and overlap between care providers. The 1992 reforms gave the 284 municipalities, previously having the authority for social care, the main role for the care of older people, including nursing homes, long-term medical care and social welfare services. The municipalities were also given the financial responsibility for patients who remained in acute hospitals after their treatment had ended, providing a financial incentive to ensure timely discharge. The 23 counties, previously responsible for health care, were given the main role for the provision of acute care (Thorslund and Parker, 1994). These arrangements have converted the health/social care division into one between acute care and long-term care, which are sequential stages in the provision of care, reflecting a logic derived from vertical integration. Thus, the Swedish reforms offer a means of achieving vertical integration within long-term care, but a boundary remains with the acute sector. Wiener (1996) has suggested that, driven by both quality of care and cost concerns, there is an increasing interest in strategies that integrate acute care and long-term care services. However, there are major barriers to the effective implementation of any such approach to apparently seamless care. For example, the integration of long-term care with the more prestigious and powerful acute care services could further disadvantage long-term care in terms of resource allocation. In practice, therefore, the achievement of integration may be less the pursuit of seamlessness than the definition of boundaries which most effectively minimise negative incentives, with mechanisms introduced to make any such boundary as permeable as possible.

Interestingly, the 1997 Mental Health Green Paper *Developing Effective Partnerships in Mental Health* (Cm 3555, 1997) reflects more of the vertical integration arguments. Four options were proposed: the creation of a mental health and social care authority; the development of a single authority for mental health services; the creation of a joint health and social care body; and agreed delegation between agencies. Each involves a greater degree of vertical integration by bringing together in closer organisational contact the different stages in the production of mental health care. It is noticeable that the proposals have the potential to bring together two elements which have been found to be associated with effective partnerships, namely the presence of appropriate financial incentives for partnerships and the presence of explicit guidance from the centre on appropriate models and procedures (Huxley et al., 1996). Although these arguments were posed in the specific context of the provision of mental health services, there is no reason why the logic of achieving greater integration in this way should not be extended to other client groups who require long-term care. Mental health services appear to be the easiest area in which to attempt such a move in the first instance, since the balance of both expenditure and organisational responsibility, arising from such approaches as the Care Programme Approach (Department of Health, 1990), provide a basis for defining which agency might take the lead role. Such arrangements might be harder to define in the case of older people, where both health and social care agencies have a major commitment and investment.

Conclusion

There would appear to be complementary requirements in health care and in social care, and in processes such as assessment, which offer real opportunities for the development of new service models. Secondary health care services, such as geriatric medicine and old age psychiatry, increasingly see their patients receiving care in their own homes or in nursing homes, giving rise to developments such as the community geriatrician (British Geriatrics Society, 1994) and more community-oriented approaches in old age psychiatry (Lindesay, 1991; Dening, 1992). Similarly, social services departments will need to develop more differentiated approaches to care management, in particular intensive care management, where the natural links for case-finding and access to expertise for assessment, support and rehabilitation are with secondary health care. Such links, bringing together service elements at different stages in the production process, can be seen as a form of vertical integration, a means of achieving a more effective partnership between health and social care.

References

Applebaum, R.A. and Austin, C.D. (1990) *Long-Term Care Case Management: Design and Evaluation*, Springer, New York.

Applegate, W.B., Miller, S.T., Graney, M.J., Elam, J.T., Burns, R. and Akins, D.E. (1990) A randomized, controlled trial of a geriatric assessment unit in a community rehabilitation hospital, *New England Journal of Medicine*, 322, 22, 1572-8.

Audit Commission (1997) *The Coming of Age: Improving Care Services for Older People*, Audit Commission, London.

Bach, D., Bach, M., Böhmer, F., Frühwald, T. and Grile, B. (1995) Reactivating occupational therapy: a method to improve cognitive performance in geriatric patients, *Age and Ageing*, 24, 3, 222-6.

Banerjee, S. and Macdonald, A.J.D. (1996) Mental disorder in an elderly home care population: associations with health and social service use, *British Journal of Psychiatry*, 168, 6, 750-56.

Banerjee, S., Shamash, K., Macdonald, A.J.D. and Mann, A.H. (1996) Randomised controlled trial of effect of intervention by psychogeriatric team on depression in frail elderly people at home, *British Medical Journal*, 313, 1058-61.

Beardshaw, V. (1988) *Last on the List: Community Services for People with Physical Disabilities*, Research Report No. 3, King's Fund Institute, London.

Bowns, I., Challis, D. and Tong, M.S. (1991) Case finding in elderly people: validation of a postal questionnaire, *British Journal of General Practice*, 41, 344, 100-104.

British Geriatrics Society (1994) *Guidelines for the Role of Community Geriatrician*, British Geriatrics Society, London.

Brocklehurst, J.C., Carty, M.H., Leeming, J.T. and Robinson, J.M. (1978) Care of the elderly: medical screening of old people accepted for residential care, *The Lancet*, ii, 141-142.

Buglass, D. (1993) *Assessment and Care Management: A Scottish Overview of Impending Change*, Community Care in Scotland Discussion Paper No. 2, Social Work Research Centre, University of Stirling.

Challis, D.J. (1994) *Implementing Caring for People: Care Management: Factors Influencing its Development in the Implementation of Community Care*, Department of Health, London.

Challis, D.J., Darton, R.A., Johnson, L., Stone, M. and Traske, K.J. (1995) *Care Management and Health Care of Older People: The Darlington Community Care Project*, Arena, Aldershot.

Challis, D.J., von Abendorff, R., Brown, P. and Chesterman, J.F. (1997) Care management and dementia: an evaluation of the Lewisham Intensive Case Management Scheme, in S. Hunter (ed.) *Research Highlights in Social Work 31. Dementia: Challenges and New Directions*, Jessica Kingsley Publishers, London.

Cm 849 (1989) *Caring for People: Community Care in the Next Decade and Beyond*, HMSO, London.

Cm 3555 (1997) *Developing Partnerships in Mental Health*, The Stationery Office, London.

Dalton, J.R. and Busch, K.D. (1995) Depression. The missing diagnosis in the elderly, *Home Healthcare Nurse*, 13, 5, 31-5.

Darton, R.A., Netten, A.P. and Brown, P. (1997) A longitudinal study of admissions to residential and nursing home care following the community care reforms, paper presented at the British Society of Gerontology Conference, Bristol, 19-21 September 1997.

Dening, T. (1992) Community psychiatry of old age: a UK perspective, *International Journal of Geriatric Psychiatry*, 7, 10, 757-66.

Department of Health (1990) *Health and Social Services Development: "Caring for People". The Care Programme Approach for People with a Mental Illness Referred to the Specialist Psychiatric Services*, HC(90)23/LASSL(90)11, Department of Health, London.

Department of Health (1992) *Community Care*, LASSL(92)8, Department of Health, London.

Department of Health (1993) *Monitoring and Development: Assessment Special Study*, Department of Health, London.

Department of Health (1994a) *Implementing Caring for People: Care Management*, Department of Health, London.

Department of Health (1994b) *Hospital Discharge Workbook: A Manual on Hospital Discharge Practice*, Department of Health, London.

Department of Health (1995a) *NHS Responsibilities for Meeting Continuing Health Care Needs*, HSG(95)8, LAC(95)5, Department of Health, London.

Department of Health (1995b) *Community Care Plans from 1996/97*, LAC(95)19, Department of Health, London.

Department of Health (1997) *Better Services for Vulnerable People*, EL(97)62, CI(97)24, Department of Health, London.

Department of Health and the Welsh Office (1989) *General Practice in the National Health Service: A New Contract*, Department of Health, London, and the Welsh Office.

Donald, I.P., Baldwin, R.N. and Bannerjee, M. (1995) Gloucester Hospital-at-Home: a randomized controlled trial, *Age and Ageing*, 24, 5, 434-9.

Evans, L.K., Yurkow, J. and Siegler, E.L. (1995) The CARE Program: a nurse-managed collaborative outpatient program to improve function of frail older people, *Journal of the American Geriatrics Society*, 43, 10, 1155-60.

Fairhurst, K., Blair, M., Cutting, J., Featherstone, M., Hayes, B., Howarth, M., Rose, D. and Stanley, I. (1996) The quality of hospital discharge: a survey of discharge arrangements for the over-65s, *International Journal for Quality in Health Care*, 8, 2, 167-74.

Farnworth, M.G., Kenny, P. and Shiell, A. (1994) The costs and effects of early discharge in the management of fractured hip, *Age and Ageing*, 23, 3, 190-94.

Garraway, W.M., Akhtar, A.J., Hockey, L. and Prescott, R.J. (1980) Management of acute stroke in the elderly: follow-up of a controlled trial, *British Medical Journal*, 281, 827-9.

Gibbon, B. and Thompson, A. (1992) The role of the nurse in rehabilitation, *Nursing Standard*, 6, 36, 32-5.

Gladman, J., Forster, A. and Young, J. (1995) Hospital- and home-based rehabilitation after discharge from hospital for stroke patients: analysis of two trials, *Age and Ageing*, 24, 1, 49-53.

Harada, N., Chiu, V., Fowler, E., Lee, M. and Reuben, D.B. (1995) Physical therapy to improve functioning of older people in residential care facilities, *Physical Therapy*, 75, 9, 830-38.

Hastings, M. (1997) The role of the physiotherapist in continuing care, in M.J. Denham (ed.) *Continuing Care for Older People*, Stanley Thornes, Cheltenham.

Hollingworth, W., Todd, C., Parker, M., Roberts, J.A. and Williams, R. (1993) Cost analysis of early discharge after hip fracture, *British Medical Journal*, 307, 903-6.

House of Commons Health Committee (1995) *Long-Term Care: NHS Responsibilities for Meeting Continuing Health Care Needs*, Volume 1, First Report, Session 1995-96, HC19-I, HMSO, London.

Huxley, P.J., Hughes, J. and Challis, D.J. (1996) *Effective Partnerships in Mental Health: A Review of the Literature*, Personal Social Services Research Unit and Mental Health Social Work Research Unit, University of Manchester, Manchester.

Ineichen, B. (1994) Managing demented old people in the community: a review, *Family Practice*, 11, 2, 210-15.

Isaacs, B. (1981) Is geriatrics a specialty?, in T. Arie (ed.) *Health Care of the Elderly*, Croom Helm, London.

Jorm, A.F., Henderson, S., Scott, R., Mackinnon, A.J., Korten, A.E. and Christensen, H. (1993) The disabled elderly living in the community: care received from family and formal services, *Medical Journal of Australia*, 158, 6, 383-8.

Lindesay, J. (ed.) (1991) *Working Out: Setting up and Running Community Psychogeriatric Teams*, Research and Development for Psychiatry, London.

Martin, F., Oyewole, A. and Moloney, A. (1994) A randomized controlled trial of a high support hospital discharge team for elderly people, *Age and Ageing*, 23, 3, 228-34.

Mulley, G.P. (1994) Principles of rehabilitation, *Reviews in Clinical Gerontology*, 4, 61-9.

National Health Service and Community Care Act 1990 (1990 c. 19) HMSO, London.

Nolan, M. (1997) Gerontological nursing: professional priority or eternal Cinderella?, *Ageing and Society*, 17, 4, 447-60.

Øvretveit, J. (1993) *Coordinating Community Care: Multidisciplinary Teams and Care Management*, Open University Press, Buckingham.

Peet, S.M., Castleden, C.M., Potter, J.F. and Jagger, C. (1994) The outcome of a medical examination for applicants to Leicestershire homes for older people, *Age and Ageing*, 23, 1, 65-8.

Peet, S.M., Castleden, C.M., McGrother, C.W. and Duffin, H.M. (1996) The management of urinary incontinence in residential and nursing homes for older people, *Age and Ageing*, 25, 2, 139-43.

Rockwood, K., Stolee, P. and McDowell, I. (1996) Factors associated with institutionalization of older people in Canada: testing a multifactorial definition of frailty, *Journal of the American Geriatrics Society*, 44, 5, 578-82.

Rubenstein, L.V., Calkins, D.R., Greenfield, S., Jette, A.M., Meenan, R.F., Nevins, M.A., Rubenstein, L.Z., Wasson, J.H. and Williams, M.E. (1988) Health status assessment for elderly patients. Report of the Society of General Internal Medicine Task Force on Health Assessment, *Journal of the American Geriatrics Society*, 37, 6, 562-9.

Rubenstein, L.Z., Aronow, H.U., Schloe, M., Steiner, A., Alessi, C.A, Yuhas, K.E., Gold, M., Kemp, M., Raube, K., Nisenbaum, R., Stuck, A. and Beck, J.C. (1994) A home-based geriatric assessment, follow-up and health promotion program: design, methods, and baseline findings from a 3-year randomized clinical trial, *Aging Clinical and Experimental Research*, 6, 2, 105-20.

Russell Hodgson, C. (1997) *"Its All Good Practice": Evaluating Practice-based Care Management in Greenwich*, Tomlinson Project No. 58, October 1994 - March 1997, South East Institute of Public Health, Tunbridge Wells.

Scottish Borders Council Social Work Department (1997) *Achieving Care Together: A Review of Assessment and Care Management in Scottish Borders. Ten Options for Change*, Scottish Borders Council, Newtown St Boswells.

Sharma, S.S., Aldous, J. and Robinson, M. (1994) Assessing applicants for Part III accommodation: is a formal clinical assessment worthwhile?, *Public Health*, 108, 2, 91-7.

Silverman, M., Musa, D., Martin, D.C., Lave, J.R., Adams, J. and Ricci, E.M. (1995) Evaluation of outpatient geriatric assessment: a randomized multi-site trial, *Journal of the American Geriatrics Society*, 43, 7, 733-40.

Social Services Inspectorate and Social Work Services Group (SSI/SWSG) (1991) *Care Management and Assessment: Managers' Guide*, HMSO, London.

Social Services Inspectorate (SSI) (1995) *The Social Services Contribution to the Rehabilitation of Older People*, Report of Conference, July 1995, Social Services Inspectorate, London.

Social Services Inspectorate (SSI) (1997) *Better Management, Better Care*, The Sixth Annual Report of the Chief Inspector Social Services Inspectorate 1996/97, The Stationery Office, London.

Stuck, A.E., Siu, A.L., Wieland, G.D., Adams, J. and Rubenstein, L.Z. (1993) Comprehensive geriatric assessment: a meta-analysis of controlled trials, *The Lancet*, 342, 1032-6.

Stuck, A.E., Zwahlen, H.G., Neuenschwander, B.E., Meyer Schweizer, R.A., Bauen, G. and Beck, J.C. (1995) Methodologic challenges of randomized controlled studies on in-home comprehensive geriatric assessment: the EIGER project. Evaluation of In-Home Geriatric Health Visits in Elderly Residents, *Aging Clinical and Experimental Research*, 7, 3, 218-23.

Thorslund, M. and Parker, M.G. (1994) Care of the elderly in the changing Swedish welfare state, in D.J. Challis, B.P. Davies and K.J. Traske (eds) *Community Care: New Agendas and Challenges from the UK and Overseas*, Arena, Aldershot.

Townsend, J., Piper, M., Frank, A.O., Dyer, S., North, W.R.S. and Meade, T.W. (1988) Reduction in hospital readmission stay of elderly patients by a community based hospital discharge scheme: a randomised controlled trial, *British Medical Journal*, 297, 544-47.

Tsuji, I., Whalen, S. and Finucane, T.E. (1995) Predictors of nursing home placement in community-based long-term care, *Journal of the American Geriatrics Society*, 43, 7, 761-6.

Victor, C.R. and Vetter, N.J. (1988) Rearranging the deckchairs on the Titanic: failure of an augmented home help scheme after discharge to reduce the length of stay in hospital, *Archives of Gerontology and Geriatrics*, 7, 83-91.

Walker, G. (1995) Therapists and nurses in older people's rehabilitation: unmet role performance expectations, *British Journal of Therapy and Rehabilitation*, 2, 1, 9-12.

Warren, M.W. (1946) Care of the chronic aged sick, *The Lancet*, i, 841-3.

Waters, K. (1987) The role of nursing in rehabilitation care, *Science and Practice*, 5, 3, 17-21.

Waters, K. (1996) Rehabilitation, in L. Wade and K. Waters (eds) *A Textbook of Gerontological Nursing: Perspectives on Practice*, Baillière Tindall, London.

Waters, K. and Luker, K.A. (1996) Staff perspectives on the role of the nurse in rehabilitation wards for elderly people, *Journal of Clinical Nursing*, 5, 2, 103-14.

Webb, A.L. and Wistow, G. (1986) *Planning, Need and Scarcity: Essays on the Personal Social Services*, Allen and Unwin, London.

Wiener, J.M. (1996) Managed care and long-term care: the integration of financing and services, *Generations*, 20, 2, 47-52.

Williamson, J., Stokoe, I.H., Gray, S., Fisher, M., Smith, A., McGhee, A. and Stephenson, E. (1964) Old people at home. Their unreported needs, *The Lancet*, i, 1117-20.

Wright, W.B. (1983) Rehabilitation, in J.M. Graham and H.M. Hodkinson (eds) *Effective Geriatric Medicine: The Special Work of Physicians in Geriatric Medicine*, Harrogate Seminar Reports 7, Department of Health and Social Security, London.

Young, J. (1994) Community care allows patients to reach their full potential, *British Medical Journal*, 309, 1356-7.

Young, J.B. and Forster, A. (1992) The Bradford community stroke trial: results at six months, *British Medical Journal*, 304, 1085-9.

Author Index